SUPER-POWE
IMMUNITY
Starts in the
GUT

T0009386

"A well-researched and thorough look at healing our gut and the importance of healing the gut first. Dr. Cook details how when our microbial world is off in our gut, it can affect our entire immune system. She helps us find the right probiotics and prebiotics for our specific health issue. She also details the best diets, foods, and practices for getting the gut back in order. This book is a valuable contribution to the burgeoning field of understanding the relationship of the immune system and the gut."

VIR MCCOY, AUTHOR OF *LIBERATING YOURSELF FROM LYME*
AND *HEALING THERAPIES FOR LONG COVID*

"Reminding us of our body's amazing capacity to heal and self-regulate, Dr. Cook applies her years of experience and research to clearly yet simply explain how our immune system, in synergistic collaboration with the microbiotic inhabitants within our body, arms our defense and ability to absorb vital life-sustaining nutrients. Discover practical magic-bullet foods as well as prebiotic and probiotic remedies that will restore and maintain healthy microbial balance to create and optimize resilience and increase wellness and vitality. A highly recommended addition to your well-being toolbox."

HEATHER DAWN GODFREY, PGCE, BSC, AUTHOR OF
HEALING WITH ESSENTIAL OILS AND
ESSENTIAL OILS FOR THE WHOLE BODY

SUPER-POWERED IMMUNITY
Starts in the
GUT

Michelle Schoffro Cook, Ph.D., DNM

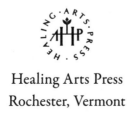

Healing Arts Press
Rochester, Vermont

Healing Arts Press
One Park Street
Rochester, Vermont 05767
www.HealingArtsPress.com

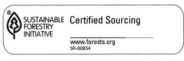

Text stock is SFI certified

Healing Arts Press is a division of Inner Traditions International

Note to the reader: *This book is intended as an informational guide. The remedies,
approaches, and techniques described herein are meant to supplement, and not to be a
substitute for, professional medical care or treatment. They should not be used to treat
a serious ailment without prior consultation with a qualified health care professional.*

Cataloging-in-Publication Data for this title is available from the Library of Congress

ISBN 978-1-64411-740-8 (print)
ISBN 978-1-64411-741-5 (ebook)

Printed and bound in the United States by Lake Book Manufacturing, LLC
The text stock is SFI certified. The Sustainable Forestry Initiative® program
promotes sustainable forest management.

10 9 8 7 6 5 4 3 2 1

Text design and layout by Kenleigh Manseau
This book was typeset in Garamond Premier Pro with Underland and Nobel used
as display typefaces

To send correspondence to the author of this book, mail a first-class letter to the
author c/o Inner Traditions • Bear & Company, One Park Street, Rochester, VT
05767, and we will forward the communication, or contact the author directly at
DrMichelleCook.com.

Contents

Acknowledgments

To my husband, Curtis, for your love and support, and for helping me
in too many ways to count

To Jon Graham, for your belief in this project and me as an author

To Kayla Toher and everyone at Inner Traditions who contributed
their skills and expertise to this book

To my family, for your love and support: Michael and Deborah
Schoffro and Bobbi-Jo Meyer

Introducing the Essentials

Many years ago, when I first became interested in holistic nutrition, I read extensively about the importance of gut and bowel health. All of the natural health experts whose books I read emphasized that not only did good health begin in the gut, but it also depended on a healthy gut. While many years have passed since then, and our collective knowledge about the gut has vastly increased, our understanding of the importance of gut health to great health has only magnified.

We now know that a whopping 70 percent of our immune system resides in the gut[1] and that a healthy, microbially balanced gastrointestinal (GI) tract is one of the keys to preventing and fighting infectious diseases. While this insight is essential to great health and super-powered immunity, I could not find any books that fully captured the information about the gut–immune system connection or that packaged this critical information into an accessible format that empowers readers to transform their gut health for greater immunity.

Additionally, current books on gut health and probiotics failed to inform readers of the even more amazing research that certain probiotics can target certain types of infectious diseases to destroy them. Instead, they take a shotgun approach informing readers to take a probiotic pill to boost gut health. While that's a start, it doesn't come close to maximizing the bacteria- and virus-killing ability of certain probiotics. This insight is not just nice to know but something that could mean the difference between life and death.

Shocked that this approach of using specific probiotics to target disease-causing microbes is still virtually unknown among medical professionals, barely known even among natural health professionals, and largely unmentioned in books on gut health or healthy immunity, I knew that I had to arm readers with this exciting information and the tools they needed to use it for maximum immunity and also to maximize their results in targeting infections using nature's most powerful anti-infectious weapons, which include probiotics. This insight has never been more critical to have at your fingertips. The shotgun approach largely used with probiotics may be fine if you have great health, but only modestly effective if you're trying to overcome infectious diseases or build super-powered immunity.

Super-Powered Immunity Starts in the Gut is the book I wished I could read but couldn't find because it did not appear to exist. *Super-Powered Immunity Starts in the Gut* delivers exciting, potentially life-saving research about particular strains that are demonstrating effectiveness against even the most drug-resistant health conditions like methicillin-resistant *Staphylococcus aureus* (MRSA), *C. difficile,* and other serious life-threatening infections and, of course, against lesser infections that need to be addressed to help you stay strong, healthy, and avoid illnesses that can be costly in terms of time off work, lost productivity at home, and quality of life.

I've attempted to share this critical information in a practical, hands-on, empowering book to help you take charge of your gut health and transform your immune system, even if you don't have any background in science or knowledge about how the body works or insight about probiotics. It includes quizzes to help you assess your gut health status, whether or not you might have an imbalanced microbiome—don't worry if you don't know what a microbiome is. I'll explain it shortly, but you really don't need to know the terminology to benefit from the advice I share throughout *Super-Powered Immunity Starts in the Gut.* Through self-assessment questionnaires, I'll help you determine whether you might suffer from excessive gut permeability that gives dangerous microbes access to your blood or other gut-related issues that may be interfering with your immune system health and overall health.

Perhaps most importantly, I'll arm you with powerful and natural ways to heal the gut, restore microbial balance, and boost your immune system against pathogenic invaders. You'll discover how to use probiotics and prebiotics, along with foods, herbs, and other remedies and lifestyle changes, to heal your gut for supercharged immune health, which in turn, is the foundation for feeling great and living life to the fullest.

Super-Powered Immunity Starts in the Gut will also teach you what to do immediately if you're taking antibiotics or have already suffered gut or immune system damage from having done so, or if you suspect that you might be suffering from the silent damage of antibiotic use and wish to prevent serious problems down the road.

Armed with the tools showcased in *Super-Powered Immunity Starts in the Gut,* you'll learn how to transform your gut health and boost your immunity against infectious diseases at the same time.

In chapter 1, "The Amazing Gut–Immune System Connection," you'll discover what superbugs are and why addressing them at the gut level is critical to superior immunity. You'll learn how the gut and immune system are connected and how beneficial bacteria even help to regulate the immune system cells that attack harmful disease, as well as how to minimize the gut-health destroyers that could be wreaking havoc on your immune system without your awareness.

In chapter 2, "Do You Have the Guts for Super-Powered Immunity?," I'll share with you the signs and symptoms of gut microbial imbalances, as well as a condition in which the gut becomes excessively leaky due to damage to the gut lining. You'll conduct self-assessment quizzes to help you determine whether you might be experiencing these health issues or whether you might have a condition known as candidiasis, or candida overgrowth. By first understanding the signs of specific gut issues, you'll be better able to address them with the information I'll share in the chapters that follow.

In chapter 3, "Probiotic-Powered Immunity," you'll learn the little-known secrets of probiotics that go well beyond popping a daily pill, including the main families of beneficial bacteria and yeasts, the parts of your gut they colonize, and how they work to ensure your survival.

One of the most exciting things you'll discover in chapter 4, "The Pro-Powered Superheroes against Colds, Flu, and Superbugs," is that probiotics are demonstrating the incredible capacity to kill harmful infectious bacteria and viruses. Bacteria fighting bacteria sounds more like science fiction than science fact, but you'll learn how to arm yourself with this amazing knowledge to keep harmful microbes at bay.

If you've been hearing about the healing benefits of fermented foods, you'll love chapter 5, "Fermented Foods: The Nearly Forgotten Wisdom of Our Ancestors," where you're sure to learn some new and exciting things about the incredible gut-healing and immune-boosting properties of many cultured delights.

In chapter 6, "The Seven-Step Plan," you'll discover the seven-pronged approach to superior gut health, powerful digestion, and ways to transform your immune system for super-powered immunity. You'll learn the best remedies to overcome harmful microbes, forty-five ways to incorporate more of them into your diet, how to beat a candida infection and restore a leaky gut, and everything you need to know to boost your gut health and immunity.

In chapter 7, "The Guts for Super Immunity—for Life," you'll find more strategies for boosting your microbiome for life.

1

The Amazing Gut–Immune System Connection

In this chapter, you'll discover:

- the gut–immune system connection;
- superbugs: what they are, and why new strategies for addressing them are critical;
- how a healthy gut can transform your immune system;
- the little-known tissue in your gut and body that plays a role in regulating the immune system;
- how immune cells known as T cells and the bacteria that help to regulate them may be the secret to great health and a long life;
- the gut-health destroyers and how to minimize their damage; and
- much more.

Your body is a wondrous creation that is more intelligent and powerful than many people realize. It extracts macro- and micronutrients alike from the wonderful (and sometimes weird) concoctions of foods we feed it. It extends a figurative lending hand to beneficial microbes that reside in your gut, offering them a portion of these newly acquired macronutrients from our meals in exchange for their proliferation and healing assistance. And that's just the beginning of the incredible ways your body extracts nutrients to support every other function in your body, of which the immune system is one of the most amazing bodily systems.

YOUR IMMUNE SYSTEM AND HOW IT KEEPS YOU HEALTHY

Your body attacks and kills foreign invaders that may have hijacked the foods we eat, destroying them in an acid bath before they gain further access to our body where they would otherwise do more damage. It draws both macro- and micronutrients through walls of the intestines where they gain direct access to the blood, which then ferries them throughout your body to repair cellular and tissue damage, quell inflammation, and construct healthy new cells that can perform healing duties anywhere in your body. And those are just a few of the incredible tasks performed by our digestive system. You'll soon discover how your gut is far more impressive than you've ever imagined.

The immune system is a powerful multiline defense system our body uses to protect us against foreign invaders of all kinds, as well as illness. As old as the first human ancestors on the planet, the fact that we are here at this time proves just how powerful the immune system is. After all, our ancestors faced many bacterial, viral, or other microbial threats and yet, they survived without pharmaceutical drug intervention. Most drugs are only several years old, and even the oldest ones only date back to the last hundred or so years. After all, the system we accept as modern medicine is itself only one to two hundred years old. That's a drop in the bucket of time and the overall history of humans on the planet.

Your immune system assesses whether foreign substances floating around in your body are a threat to your health and, if so, readies the troops for attack. In this capacity, the "troops" are various components of your immune system, including five main ones:

The Tonsils and Thymus Gland: The tonsils are a mass of tissue at the back of your throat while the thymus is a gland in your upper chest. They are responsible for producing antibodies—substances that are combatants against foreign invaders in your body.

The Lymphatic System: A vast network of lymph nodes and vessels that carry lymphatic fluid, nutrients, and waste products between your bodily tissues and bloodstream. The lymph nodes filter the fluid that passes between them, capturing viruses, bacteria, and other foreign invaders, which are then destroyed by white blood cells known as lymphocytes that are also the body's soldiers against infectious diseases.

Bone Marrow: The bone marrow is a soft tissue that is primarily located inside the larger bones of your body, including the arms, legs, vertebrae, and pelvis. While we think of our bones as fairly static and inanimate, in reality, they are involved in different processes of the body, including playing an important part of our immune system. The red marrow produces red and white blood cells. The yellow marrow helps in the production of white blood cells. These blood cells attack a wide range of foreign invaders in the body.

The Spleen: The spleen is an organ on the left side of your abdomen. It filters the blood by removing old or damaged cells while also destroying bacteria and other foreign invaders that may otherwise compromise your health.

White Blood Cells: Made in the bone marrow, these cells attack and destroy organisms, such as bacteria, viruses, or other microbes, that could threaten your health.[1]

Chances are you don't give your immune system much consideration when you're healthy. Few people do. It's really only when people get sick or worry about something that's "going around" that they want to ensure their immune system is working optimally. That's in part because your immune system is constantly working and doing such an impressive job that you don't even notice its many battles with foreign infectious invaders because it overcomes them and you stay healthy. And it does all this with little thought given to it. Most people would be shocked to know just how hard their immune system works on a regular basis to keep them healthy. Here are some of its many impressive functions.

Your immune system:

- fights disease-causing germs, also known as pathogens, which include bacteria, fungi, and viruses;
- removes pathogens from your body;
- recognizes and neutralizes harmful substances from the environment; and
- fights disease-causing changes in the body, including cancer cells.[2]

Your immune system assesses the proteins on the surfaces of various types of microbes, including bacteria, fungi, and viruses, since they differ from your own cells and tissues. These proteins, known as antigens, bind to the immune system cells, triggering a series of processes that launch the immune system's responses.

When your body comes into contact with a disease-causing microbe for the first time, it stores information about it and how to best fight it so your immune system is faster and more efficient should it ever have a showdown with the germ at a future date.[3] In other words, your immune system stores its own repository of germ-killing information.

This process and information repository also helps your body to deal with mutations of a specific microbe. While viruses and germs mutate—come back in a different form—the immune system is much more capable of fighting off the new version because it has already stored information about the microbe in its germ-killing database, so to speak. This is called "acquired immunity" or "natural immunity," which we heard so much about during the recent pandemic.

It's sort of like a germ being dressed up in a new costume, but the immune system recognizes its face and therefore knows who it is and what its weaknesses are to overcome it. Obviously, that's an oversimplification of a complex process, but it may be valuable for the sake of understanding the immune system at its core.

Maybe She's Born with It or Maybe It's Acquired?

The elements of your immune system are classified into two systems or two types, as they are also known: innate and acquired immune systems.

◊ Innate Immune System

The innate immune system is the one with which you were born. Since the day you were born your immune system began attacking foreign invaders to keep you healthy. Whenever it came into contact with bacteria, fungi, viruses, or other pathogens, your immune system acted quickly to engulf the invader using its cells known as phagocytes. These frontline immune system cells immediately sprang into action to kill harmful microbes to keep you safe and healthy. The innate immune system is also called the nonspecific immune system because it functions in a general manner and doesn't need to know the identity of the virus or other microbe with which it is dealing to begin immediately attacking it.

But don't be fooled: it may be a generalized system, but it is still highly effective at killing harmful microbes. Its natural killer cells and phagocytes ("eating cells") work as the frontline defenses against harmful germs that largely enter the body through the digestive system or skin.[4]

◊ Acquired Immune System

Your acquired immune system, which we briefly discussed earlier, works in conjunction with the immunity you were born with by producing cells known as antibodies to protect you against foreign invaders. Antibodies are created in your body from cells known as B-lymphocytes after it has been exposed to a specific invader. If during the pandemic you came into contact with the SARS-CoV2 virus that caused COVID-19, your body's B-lymphocytes worked to create antibodies to help you stay healthy or to prevent serious illness or death. You may recall many people saying they had natural immunity and that such powerful immunity needed to be factored into policy decisions. They were referring to their immune system having come into contact with that particular virus and that they now have the immune cells known as antibodies that help to protect them against reinfection and even against new variants of the virus. Acquired immunity often protects your body against new variants of the same disease.

The acquired immune system is in constant flux as it adapts throughout your lifetime to new and varied microbial challenges, including bacterial, fungal, or viral threats. As it meets these new challenges, it develops antibodies against them and stores the information on how to battle and win whenever it comes into contact with them again.

Antibodies can take a few days for the immune system to create, but that doesn't mean your immune system is waiting to attack a foreign invader. As soon as it notices an invader, it immediately begins attacking it. Once it recognizes the invader as something it has come into contact with before, its antibodies assist your immune system in overcoming the threat. And they help ensure that you're far less likely to deal with this particular infection in the future.

The Growing Superbug Dilemma

You've probably been hearing a lot about superbugs in recent times but may be wondering what exactly they are. Superbugs are strains of bacteria, fungi, parasites, and viruses that are resistant to most of the antibiotic drugs (in the case of bacteria) or other medications that are commonly used to treat the infections caused by these microbes. Depending on the specific bacteria, fungus, or virus involved, they can cause a range of infections, some of which include pneumonia or other respiratory infections like MRSA, skin infections, urinary tract infections,[5] gonorrhea, or blood infections known as sepsis. There are many resistant microbes, such as bacteria that are increasingly becoming a threat, some of which include: *Staphylococcus aureus*, *Klebsiella pneumonia*, *Escherichia coli* (*E. coli*), and *Clostridium difficile*. Don't worry if you can't remember or pronounce their names, as it isn't necessary to ramp up your immune system to help fight them should you come into contact with them in the future or if you've already come into contact with them.

Resistance, drug resistance, or antimicrobial resistance, all of which are different names for the same phenomenon, occurs over time. And, while it can happen naturally, it can be hastened or exacerbated by a wide variety of things that we do, without realizing that these habits or behaviors can be worsening drug resistance. While resistance can happen with any bacteria, fungi, or viruses, we have already seen the dangers of our overuse and misuse of antibiotics (such as treating viral conditions with antibiotics that work on bacteria, not viruses) and the resulting antibiotic-resistant bacteria causing serious infections, such as MRSA (methicillin-resistant *Staphylococcus aureus*) infections.

While it may be easy to panic and live your life in fear, which sadly too many people have done, the solution to superbugs may have been right under our noses all along—in our gut. As you will soon discover, the key to super-powered immunity lies in your gut. You can set panic and fear aside in favor of building up strong gut health, which in turn can transform your immune system to help you fight off nasty infectious diseases and the harmful bacteria, fungi, or viruses behind them.

HOW YOUR GUT IS INVOLVED IN
SUPER-POWERED IMMUNITY

Now that we've briefly explored the combative powers of the immune system, let's take a quick look at the gastrointestinal (GI) tract and what happens when these two systems converge in our body, which is nothing less than pure magic.

Until fairly recently, few health practitioners realized that the gut played much of a role in healthy immunity. Over time, the research about the immune system showed that, not only does the gut play a role in a healthy immunity, but it houses approximately 70 to 80 percent of your immune system and its cells.[6,7] As a result, no discussion on immunity would be complete without a comprehensive discussion of the gut and how to transform it for super-powered immunity, yet few people, including many experts, are even aware of this connection. Before we delve into the connection, let's first take a look at your digestive system and how it works to help you stay healthy.

Digestion—The Alchemy Inside Your Body

While most people never consider their miraculous digestive system until some sort of trouble arises in the form of bloating, indigestion, heartburn, or other uncomfortable symptom, digestion is nothing short of alchemy at work within your body. The foods you eat contain protein, carbohydrates, and fats, all of which need to be broken down so the body can extract amino acids, sugars, and fatty acids, respectively. These components of food are also the building blocks of healthy cells, tissues, and organs in your body. Without them, you could not live, and with insufficient amounts of them, you wouldn't experience health. If this system breaks down, you will undoubtedly experience a decline in health and weakened immunity as your body loses its ability to maintain and build healthy new cells, tissues, and organs due to insufficient nutrients.

The food you eat, provided it is healthy, also contains vitamins, minerals, enzymes (specialized proteins that help perform certain chemical processes in your body), phytonutrients (plant nutrients that help to keep you healthy), and, ideally, probiotics (beneficial microbes) as well. Whenever I tell people this fundamental nutritional information, inevitably I find someone who says that these foundational nutrients are not actually necessary. I can't help but chuckle because the Oxford Dictionary defines a vitamin as "any of a group of organic compounds which *are essential* for normal growth and nutrition and are required in small quantities in the diet because they cannot be synthesized in the body."[8] Minerals are the inorganic substances found in food that are also essential to the functioning of the body and include such elements as calcium, magnesium, iron, boron, and others.

Your GI system comprises many organs, including the mouth, salivary glands (located in the mouth), stomach, small intestines, large intestines, liver, gall bladder, pancreas, and others. The average person's GI tract is about twenty feet long and processes approximately twenty-five tons of food over his or her lifetime, while also conducting other essential functions in the body. That's an astounding feat by any measure.

Digestion begins the moment you start eating; chewing stimulates the secretion of digestive juices in the salivary glands in your mouth, where it begins breaking down the starchy components of your food. That's why chewing your food is imperative to healthy digestion.

After swallowing your food, it passes through the esophagus, which is a tube that joins the mouth and the stomach. The food then sits for about twenty to thirty minutes in the stomach mixing with the enzymes in the food (this applies to uncooked foods only as the enzymes found in food are destroyed through the cooking process) and the digestive juices secreted in your mouth. At that point, the food is hit with an acid bath known as hydrochloric acid, which helps to break down protein foods into amino acids.

The food then passes into the intestines where nutrients are absorbed through fingerlike protrusions known as villi, which help to aid the absorption of the nutrients directly into the bloodstream, where the nutrients will travel via the blood to the places in the body that they are most needed. For example, calcium often travels via the blood to the bones or nerves while magnesium may travel to your muscles, nerves, or other parts of the body where this "relaxation" nutrient is needed. This is an oversimplification because nutrients may be needed everywhere but are especially in demand in certain parts of the body.

Of course, there are other aspects of digestion, but these are the most critical for our discussion of the gut and its connection to the immune system.

The Gut-Immune System Connection

Our digestive tract is one of the main contact points for our external environment and is often overloaded with foods or beverages that may contain toxic substances or pathogens like bacteria, fungi, and viruses. It also intakes and processes food (or supplements) breaking it down into its foundational nutrients so they can become the building blocks of our cells. We're frequently coming into contact with harmful microbes in our food, yet we rarely ever get food poisoning because our immune system works hard to ensure that we don't. However, periodically some particularly troublesome microbes find their way into our bodies, making our immune systems work extra hard.

On those occasions when you may have eaten something that was "off" you've probably experienced the gut–immune system link without even realizing it as your gut fought off *Escherichia coli* (*E.coli*) or another microbe that may have contaminated your food, causing nausea, abdominal discomfort, diarrhea, and other symptoms.

Researchers discovered what is known as gut-associated lymphoid tissue (GALT), which in itself is a critical component of the immune system and warrants discussion as one of the main lines of defense against foreign invaders. The gut contains a massive number of immune system cells, collectively known as GALT. Made up of immune system cells known as B and T cells, macrophages, and other cells, this mass of tissue works as an early line of defense against foreign invaders that may find their way into your body.[9]

GALT includes the lymphoid tissue associated with the gut, including the tonsils, Peyer's patches, lamina propria of the gastrointestinal tract, and appendix.[10] Here's a quick overview of these components of the GALT:

Tonsils: Your tonsils are two small oval masses found at the back of your throat.

Peyer's Patches: Peyer's patches are tissue that is found in your small intestines.

Lamina Propria of the GI Tract: A thin layer of connective tissue beneath the mucous membranes lining the gut.[11]

Lymphocytes in the intestinal surfaces: Nearly colorless cells found in the blood, lymph, and lymphoid tissues;[12]

Appendix: A tubular projection attached to the large intestines[13]

It's not necessary to remember all the different components or their names, or even how to pronounce them, but it is valuable to understand how integral this tissue is to your immune system and to keeping you healthy, and maybe even slowing down aging and helping you to live longer too.

The GALT plays an important role in the immune system to help it recognize food, cells, and healthy bacteria so as to not wage war against them.[14] It also plays an imperative role in rousing the immune system troops to battle against infectious microbes while assessing when to relax these efforts.[15]

Researchers at the Massachusetts Institute of Technology Center for Microbiome Informatics and Therapeutics found that the gut even plays an important role in controlling immune system functioning. While our understanding of the microbes in our gut is still in its infancy, these researchers discovered that these gut microbes and immune system cells talk to each other. T cells, which are created in the bone marrow, play a role in either rousing the immune system to fight or pumping the brakes when the battle is over or no longer needed.[16] This balance of duties is necessary to ensure that we remain healthy by the immune system being able to fight off infection but not function excessively to the point of creating a harmful cytokine storm or to attack its own tissues.

Cytokine Storms and the Probiotics that Block "Immune System Burnout"

In many viral and bacterial illnesses, including the most recent COVID-19 outbreaks, infections overactivate the immune system, creating a highly inflammatory process known as "the cytokine response." While increased immune activity can be helpful to engage the immune system, the infection hijacks the body's own immune system, causing it to overwork while wreaking havoc on healthy cells and tissues, as well as increasing the risk of death.

New frontiers in the field of probiotic research are providing hope for the possible treatment of cytokine storms, as they are also known. And the research could not be more welcome given the potentially deadly effects of this infection-induced immune system response. Research in the *Journal of the American College of Nutrition* shows that two probiotic strains, *L. gasseri* and *B. bifidum*, may reduce this inflammation and regulate the cytokine response. The probiotic supplement yielded a less inflammatory cytokine profile due to changes in the microbiome.[17]

In some conditions like inflammatory bowel diseases (IBD), Crohn's disease, psoriasis, multiple sclerosis, and rheumatoid arthritis, the T cell balance between fighting and resting can become impaired. The MIT researchers explored how bacteria might play a role on "germ-free" mice—mice that live their lives in controlled environments free of microorganisms. They found that the mice have imbalances between the two types of T cells and don't even develop the type that rouse the immune system troops to fight. It seems that having a microbiome plays a more important role than previously believed when it comes to the immune system.

The researchers also discovered that a group of bacteria known as Bacteroidetes churn out a compound called isoalloLCA that impacts T cell activity. And, perhaps most exciting, they found that people who are healthy have higher levels of the bacteria and the compound they make compared to people who are sick and that those people who live to be one hundred years or older also had higher levels of both. While the research is still early, it suggests that these beneficial bacteria may play important roles in maintaining or improving health and longevity.[18]

Other studies of germ-free mice have noted several other immune system deficiencies as a result of being devoid of beneficial microbes, including the reduction of a range of immune system cells that fight infections, as well as structural and inflammatory abnormalities. But it's not bad news: when researchers colonized the guts of the germ-free mice, they found that the GALT expanded, along with it the immune system cells needed to fight harmful infections, and the immune system and inflammatory compounds even became more regulated.[19]

There are multiple ways to boost beneficial gut colonies, including: avoiding foods, beverages, and lifestyle habits that cause their demise; probiotic supplementation; eating a range of fermented foods on a daily basis; and eating a diet rich in prebiotics (food that feeds probiotics) and that supports the conditions of a healthy gut. Don't worry if you're not familiar with these terms or concepts because we'll discuss them throughout *Super-Powered Immunity Starts in the Gut*.

THE MICROBIOME AND
THE IMMUNITY DESTROYERS

The sad reality is that due to poor food and beverage choices, antibiotic overuse or misuse, an increasingly sedentary lifestyle, and other factors that determine gut health, our gut may be in a state of distress and not conducive at all to super-powered immunity, or even basic immunity, in many cases.

We explored how the nutrients from food are extracted into the bloodstream by villi in the small intestines, but that process becomes impaired when the intestinal walls become damaged or inflamed, which largely happens as a result of poor food or beverage choices, insufficient water or fibrous foods, or excessive sugar, meat, or fat in the diet. Any or all of these habits can result in dysbiosis—an imbalance in harmful to beneficial bacteria and yeasts in the GI tract, which may result in gut inflammation and excessive permeability of the intestinal walls, which makes it easier for harmful microbes to hijack the nutrient-absorption process, giving them as well as waste products direct access to your bloodstream.

Restoring a healthy diet, healing any damage to the gut, and restoring a healthy balance of pathogenic-to-beneficial microbes is critical for healthy immunity and overall health. In chapter 6, you'll discover my seven-step plan to do all of these things.

BUILD A BETTER MICROBIOME FOR SUPER-POWERED IMMUNITY

Fortunately, our bodies inherently know how to heal our gut and to ensure a healthy microbial balance that is needed to support health and ward off disease. In most cases, as long as we provide it with the building blocks it needs to ensure a healthy microbial foundation, we can remain or become healthy. We'll discuss these building blocks in the following chapters.

We hear the term "probiotic" thrown around fairly regularly these days—can we watch a television show or flip through a magazine without seeing advertisements for probiotic-containing yogurt, supplements, or even gummies? But what exactly are these things we hear so much about?

Scientists describe probiotics as "live microorganisms that, when administered in adequate amounts, confer a health benefit on the host."[20] In other words, they are living bacteria and other microorganisms that may have the ability to improve your digestion, boost your body's ability to fight disease, strengthen immunity, and increase your body's ability to improve your health. Most people, doctors included, still use probiotics in a fairly passive and indirect manner. For example, they may recommend eating yogurt or popping a probiotic supplement and hoping that it boosts gut health and eventually improves overall immunity and health. But what if probiotics could also be used in more precise ways, such as to directly target harmful infectious diseases? A growing body of research suggests that is the direction we're heading. And the timing couldn't be better because many infectious diseases have outsmarted our drugs for killing them.

It turns out that beneficial microbes might actually be among the best tools to combat bacterial, fungal, parasitic, or viral illnesses. It's hard to imagine bacteria doing battle with other bacteria to prevent or treat infection, but that's exactly what some strains of beneficial bacteria do to help us overtake disease-causing bacteria and other microbes; they do, if we have the guts for this task. Before we delve into the exciting research, let's first take a closer look at our microbiome and how to set the foundation for this targeted, more aggressive approach to using probiotics to overcome infectious diseases.

In our modern times of fast food and junk food packed with preservatives, colors, fillers, emulsifiers, and many other toxic chemicals and other ingredients, combined with our tendency toward sedentary living, a heavy reliance on pharmaceutical drugs, extensive use of toxic-chemical-saturated personal care and household products, overwork, chronic stress, and other unhealthy lifestyle factors, our gut microbiota can easily become out of balance.

While there are many considerations for a healthy gut, which we'll discuss momentarily, microbial balance is arguably the most important because it determines whether our guts are predominantly beneficial strains of microbes or harmful, inflammation- and disease-causing ones that not only cannot fight other infectious diseases in our body, but thwart our best efforts instead.

EXPLORING THE HUMAN MICROBIOME

We tend to think of ourselves as only one being. You are you and I am me, and we are two separate individuals. It's easy to see how we have reached this conclusion. When we look in the mirror, we see only one being standing before us. And so we think that we are nothing more than that. After all, what else could we be? But thanks to extensive scientific study we now know that our bodies are made up of many microbiomes within a larger microbiome that is us. In other words, each of us is a microbiome of many different microbes. And within this microbiome there are many other smaller microbiomes.

It sounds confusing. Several years ago, scientists began studying the Human Microbiome Project (HMP). They found that each person is an ecosystem made up of millions of microorganisms. And we also have unique ecosystems in our intestines, our knees, our mouth, our tongue, on our teeth, on our wrist, and so on. Even our left hand's ecosystem differs from the ecosystem found on our right hand. These ecosystems are called microbiomes.

In the same way that no two people have the same fingerprints, we now know that no two people have the same microbiomes either. These microbiomes change depending on the things we eat, the lifestyle choices we make, and many other factors, most of which may still need to be discovered. The science surrounding microbiomes is still in its infancy, so there will likely be much more to learn over time.

Perhaps even more surprising than learning that you are not just you, but an ecosystem, is the fact that safeguarding the health of this ecosystem may be the secret to ensuring your long-term health and your body's ability to overcome disease.

Bonnie Bassler, professor of molecular biology at Princeton

University, who is best known for her research into how bacteria communicate, persuasively captured the benefits of the many beneficial bacteria that comprise our microbiome when she stated: "We mostly don't get sick. Most often bacteria are keeping us well."[21] She's right. We are made up of trillions of microorganisms, the bulk of which are primarily found in our gut. As a result, it may come as no surprise when I tell you that a large portion of our immune system begins in the gut. According to some estimates, over one trillion bacteria made up of approximately one thousand different species, weighing an estimated two pounds combined, reside in your intestines.[22]

And, as scientist Philip C. Calder stated in his study published in *BMJ Nutrition, Prevention & Health*, "the gut microbiota plays a role in educating and regulating the immune system."[23]

Beneficial microbes don't just keep us well, they are also needed to ensure our survival. They literally help us to stay alive. We could not live without the many beneficial microbes inhabiting our bodies or performing their many essential tasks.

A BALANCED MICROBIOME IS THE KEY TO STRONG IMMUNITY

Just as no fruits or vegetables, herbs, or trees can grow from toxic soil, neither can health arise from a microbiome that is overburdened with harmful microbes.

As we discussed earlier, our germ obsessions have actually backfired, resulting in imbalanced microbial landscapes, whether human or ecological. Indiscriminately waging war against all microbes in a desperate attempt to kill harmful bacteria or viruses has, in many ways, failed. The overuse of antibacterial soaps, cleaning products, and hand sanitizers that contain harsh toxic ingredients has given many microbes an opportunity to grow stronger and more resilient during the time that we have been wiping down every door handle, surface, and washing or sanitizing our hands many times a day. We have increasingly discovered that when we indiscriminately kill bacteria, we also rid ourselves of some of our best weapons against infectious diseases.

PRO-POWERED IMMUNITY—THE CORNERSTONE OF SUPER-POWERED IMMUNITY

An ever-growing body of research shows that restoring beneficial bacteria, known as probiotics, can not only strengthen our immune system, but can also help us to overcome harmful bacterial or other types of infections. Some strains of probiotics have even been found to go to battle with disease-causing viruses, to our great benefit. Of course, some strains of probiotics are better to tackle certain infections than others—a topic we'll discuss in greater detail in chapter 3.

Probiotics against Antibiotic Resistance?

What we once believed were our best weapons against bacteria-caused illness—antibiotics—we now know may be in their twilight years. While it is disheartening, we are increasingly finding that probiotics offer hope in dealing with this challenging situation and threat to our wellbeing. Probiotics show promise in the battle against harmful infections, including bacteria, fungi, and viruses. And what's more exciting is that some strains of probiotics seem to be working in conjunction with the drugs, or in some cases, even when the drugs are failing.

While some of the research is still preliminary, and in fact most of our understanding about the human microbiome is in its infancy, we can nevertheless benefit from incorporating the research into our understanding and the probiotics into our health and wellness strategy. Considering the safety and effectiveness that probiotics are demonstrating, along with the seriousness of the situation we are facing and the many health benefits of incorporating more probiotics and probiotic-rich food into our diets, probiotics can play an important role in boosting our immune health and in treating infectious conditions.

How Do Probiotics Work?

We know that antibiotic drugs work by indiscriminately killing bacteria in our intestines, but what about probiotics? Our understanding about probiotics and how they work is growing. We now understand that probiotics work against harmful microbes and the diseases they cause in at least nine ways, which include:

1. Probiotics improve the gut microbiome's stability and recovery after the microbial balance has been disrupted, such as through drugs like antibiotics or poor food choices.
2. Probiotics create antimicrobial compounds that include organic acids or bacteriocins (types of proteins that are secreted by bacteria to slow or stop the growth of other bacterial strains, such as pathogenic bacteria).
3. Probiotics improve the body's own immune response to pathogens by strengthening immunity.
4. They decrease the inflammatory response in the body, which enables the body to function in a healthier way.
5. Probiotics assist in the early programming of the immune system to result in a better-balanced immune response and a reduced risk of developing impaired immune conditions like allergies.
6. They improve the mucosal barrier in the gut and its functioning.
7. Probiotics help to regulate genetic expression for health conditions and diseases.
8. They create valuable proteins and enzymes needed by the body for optimal health.
9. They prevent harmful microbes from adhering to various locations in the body, such as in the gut wall.[24]

Over time, it is likely that we'll learn more ways that probiotics work and how they contribute to improved immunity against disease and our overall health. Regardless, we know that probiotics offer tremendous support in helping our bodies to overcome infectious disease and are therefore worth using.

THE MIRACLE OF PROBIOTICS

Using probiotics to prevent the gut microbial damage caused by antibiotics is commonplace and one of the primary ways in which probiotics are used therapeutically. But using them alongside antibiotics is really just the tip of the iceberg in using probiotics to transform both gut and immune system health. It may be a good starting point, but there are so many more immune system benefits you can reap by improving the beneficial microbes in your gut, as you'll learn throughout this book.

In fact, the use of probiotics as a direct way to boost the immune system or in the prevention or treatment of infectious diseases has hardly been considered by most medical professionals, yet the research shows that it warrants a rightful place in our immune-boosting artillery against harmful bacteria, fungi, and viruses. That's true now more than ever, particularly as our best drugs are losing their effectiveness, causing harmful side effects, and even increasing the virulence of infectious microbes, frequently resulting in superbugs.

Probiotics, on the other hand, have many positive side effects including improving our gut and overall health, reducing our susceptibility to harmful infections, and in the treatment or management of many serious chronic conditions, as you'll soon discover.

2

Do You Have the Guts for Super-Powered Immunity?

In this chapter, you'll learn:

- how your gut is the key to great health;
- the key gut issues linked to inferior immune system strength, including: dysbiosis (more harmful microbes than beneficial ones), a permeable gut membrane that gives dangerous microbes access to your blood, yeast overgrowth, and other gut-related issues; and
- a quick self-assessment quiz to determine whether you might have specific gut issues that need attention.

GREAT HEALTH BEGINS IN THE GUT

Your gut is the key to great health. It is involved in many functions that affect your whole body, right down to the health of every cell. There are many reasons why your gut is the key to transforming your overall health and immune system, but it plays key roles in digestion and nutrient absorption, reducing inflammation, maintaining a healthy body weight, allergy prevention and reduction, brain health, and, of course, healthy immunity, which you learned in chapter 1.

The Guts for Great Digestion

While it may seem obvious that improved gut health also improves digestion, it bears noting because indigestion, nausea, bloating, cramping, and other digestive troubles have become commonplace in our society and, more often than not, people pop pills with lengthy lists of side effects that do nothing to improve digestion but only mask the symptoms of gut troubles. By naturally boosting gut health, instead of covering up the symptoms with pills, you'll likely experience improved digestion and reduced symptoms of digestive distress for the long term.

The Guts for Nutrient Absorption

Nutrients that are needed to build every cell in our body are absorbed through the walls of the gut. When you eat food, it is broken down into the foundational nutrients, which, as we mentioned earlier but bears repeating, include: amino acids (from protein), fatty acids (from fats), sugars (from carbohydrates), vitamins, minerals, enzymes (specialized proteins that aid digestion and other bodily functions), and phytonutrients (which literally means plant nutrients, such as lycopene in tomatoes or proanthocyanidins in blueberries to cite only two of the possible thousands of phytonutrients in our food), among other nutrients.

When nutrients reach the gut, they travel directly across the intestinal walls into the bloodstream where they continue their journey to our bones, brain, heart, liver, or other part that needs replenishing. These amino acids, fatty acids, sugars, vitamins, minerals, and other nutrients become cells, tissues, and organs.

The Guts to Prevent and Reduce Inflammation

The gut determines whether we'll experience inflammation there or somewhere else in our bodies. That is in part due to the permeability of the intestinal walls and the bacteria that reside there.

If the gut wall becomes excessively permeable as a result of antibiotic use, excessive hormones, stress, poor diet, or other potential causes, whole food molecules (not just the nutrients) or waste matter can travel into the bloodstream.

Since these food molecules and waste materials are not supposed to be in the blood, the immune system goes on alert, attacking them, causing low-grade, ongoing inflammation that can damage the cells and tissues in the body, making them more vulnerable to illness.

The Guts for a Healthy Body Weight

Numerous studies show that the intestinal microbes of overweight and obese people were found to differ from those of lean people. In the journal *Beneficial Microbes*, researchers found that obese and overweight people tend to have a higher ratio of harmful microbes to beneficial ones.[1] Beneficial flora in our gut can help us to achieve and maintain a healthy weight in multiple ways:

1. Provide us with the energy we need through the breakdown of starches and sugars in our diet. Beneficial bacteria assist with the digestion and absorption of these carbohydrates.
2. Improve the cellular energy levels of liver and muscle cells. If the liver and muscles do not receive the energy they need to perform optimally, then they don't function adequately and cannot break down fat stores and build up muscles (which, in turn, break down fat).
3. Reduce the accumulation of fat in our tissues.

The Guts to Prevent Allergies and Allergic Reactions

According to research in the journal *International Archives of Allergy and Immunology*, some strains of beneficial bacteria exert anti-allergic effects, thereby reducing the symptoms of allergies, such as nasal congestion.[2] While allergic reactions are linked to the immune system, it's such a common concern, it warranted mention in its own right. To learn more ways to improve allergies consult my book, *Allergy-Proof Your Life*.

The Guts for a Healthy Brain

The gut is increasingly becoming known as the "second brain" among health professionals as increasing amounts of research show that gut health contributes to brain health. Some probiotics found in the gut actually function as antioxidants—nutrients that quell harmful free radicals before they can cause damage to the cells. According to research published in *BioMed Research International,* these antioxidant bacteria may exert a protective effect on cognitive function.[3]

The Guts for Healthy Immunity

As you discovered in chapter 1, you need to have a healthy gut to ensure a healthy immune system, and experts estimate that between 70 and 80 percent of our immune system cells reside in our gut. That's why we need to focus our attention on our gut health if we want to fend off harmful bacteria, fungi, and viruses. Avoiding superbugs altogether or overcoming them if we've been infected depends in large part on having a healthy gut, so it's never been more important to ensure your gut health.

A GUT IN DISTRESS IS AN IMMUNE SYSTEM IN DISTRESS

Sadly, most people suffer from signs of immune system weakness without ever realizing that an unhealthy gut lies at the root of their woes. Some people will find it difficult to accept that one of the primary reasons they get several colds or flu every year, or a more serious infectious disease, is that their gut is unhealthy. To help people understand the connection, I ask them if they ever took a course of antibiotics to treat an infection. In more cases than not, they say yes. I then ask them if they experienced signs of gut issues after taking the antibiotics to treat the other condition. Again, more often than not, people say yes. Antibiotics may work on that urinary tract, skin, or some other type of infection, but they undoubtedly throw off the beneficial microbes in the gut at the same time, causing a range of gut-related symptoms, including diarrhea. In this example, the gut–immune connection is noticeable.

Most people have taken at least one course of antibiotics in their lifetime, and many people have taken multiple courses. If you're among those who have used antibiotics, then you are probably well-versed in their side effects, which include: gastrointestinal distress, intestinal bacterial overgrowth, and the resulting diarrhea, to name a few. The side effects of antibiotics are sometimes as bad as the original health problem for which they took the drugs.

Antibiotics cause diarrhea and other gastrointestinal issues because they kill harmful bacteria and beneficial ones alike. Even if antibiotics do exactly what they are intended to do, which is to indiscriminately kill all bacteria with which they come into contact, they leave a path of microbial destruction in their wake that, ideally, needs immediate attention or attention at the first possible opportunity.

My clients were always amazed at how much better they felt when they took probiotics alongside their antibiotics. And they always returned reporting how the probiotics almost immediately stopped the antibiotic-induced diarrhea or antibiotic-related diarrhea they had experienced. That's because probiotics work to ensure a healthy gut, even when antibiotics damage the gut, indiscriminately killing both harmful and beneficial microbes alike.

Many medical doctors have begun to recognize the damage antibiotics cause to the microbiome, or at least the gut microbiome, largely due to the fact that most people suffer from diarrhea while taking a course of antibiotics. The problem is so common that it is considered a condition unto itself: antibiotic-related diarrhea. As a result of this awareness and the growing popularity of probiotics and fermented foods, a growing number of medical doctors have begun prescribing probiotic supplements and fermented foods along with their prescription for antibiotics. Unfortunately, the number of doctors doing so is still insufficient. Prescribing probiotics and fermented foods is important for those taking antibiotics to minimize the damage caused by the drugs. Of course, if your doctor has prescribed antibiotics, you should also check with him or her before altering his or her plan.

Diarrhea is one of the primary side effects of taking antibiotics, but it isn't the only issue. Because antibiotics indiscriminately kill bacteria in the gut microbiome, they destroy beneficial organisms that help to keep disease-causing bacteria in check in the intestines. Unfortunately, people can become vulnerable to other bacterial infections than those for which they initially started taking the antibiotics. Many people taking antibiotics can suffer from *Clostridium difficile* (*C. difficile*) infections. And guess one of the main symptoms of *C. difficile* infections. That's right: diarrhea. Fortunately, probiotics are also showing promise against *C. diff.*

The ever-growing body of research supports the use of probiotics alongside antibiotics. Finnish researchers studied the effectiveness of probiotic supplements to prevent antibiotic-induced diarrhea and assess the rate of *Clostridium difficile* (*C. difficile*) infections. They found a correlation between a higher dose of probiotics and a lowered incidence and duration of diarrhea experienced by people taking antibiotic drugs. They also found that participants taking probiotic supplements had fewer fevers, abdominal pain, and bloating.[4]

Californian researchers also found similar results, but their research focused on specific strains with evidence supporting their use against antibiotic-induced diarrhea and published their findings in *JAMA: The Journal of the American Medical Association.* They found that a wide variety of probiotic strains were beneficial in effectively treating the condition, including: many *Lactobacillus, Bifidobacterium, Saccharomyces, Streptococcus, Enterococcus,* and/or *Bacillus* bacteria.[5] A Swedish study found that *Lactobacillus plantarum* was also helpful.[6]

Other research showed that *Lactobacillus casei, Lactobacillus bulgaricus,* and *Streptococcus thermophilus* also cut the incidence of antibiotic-associated diarrhea by almost two-thirds.[7] Still other research found that some probiotics, including *Lactobacillus GG* and *Lactobacillus reuteri* were more effective in children than in adults and reduced the duration of hospitalization of pre-term infants.[8]

In a small study of 255 adults, scientists gave one group of people two probiotic capsules containing only two readily available probiotic strains: *L. acidophilus* and *L. casei,* while others received one capsule of a placebo and one capsule of the same probiotic blend, and still others received only placebo capsules. The researchers found that those taking two capsules of the probiotics daily had only one-third the incidence of antibiotic-associated diarrhea of those taking only placebos, or one-half the incidence of those taking the combination of probiotics and placebo pills. This study not only showed the effectiveness of the two strains taken but also that the results were dose dependent. In other words, the higher the dose people took, the fewer antibiotic-associated symptoms they experienced. In this study, the probiotics were administered for the full duration of the antibiotics, plus an additional five days. Of course, that doesn't suggest taking fistfuls of probiotics to counter the effects of antibiotics, but it does show the benefits of two pills over only one probiotic pill or none at all.[9] They also found that timing matters too. The researchers found that it was important to begin taking the probiotics immediately after starting a course of antibiotics and to continue taking them after completing the course of drugs.

And if you're still not convinced, still another study conclusively analyzed the data and found that there is good reason to be taking probiotics alongside antibiotics. In a large meta-analysis of thirty-four randomized, double-blind, placebo-controlled studies including 4,138 people, researchers concluded that taking probiotics along with antibiotics prevents the antibiotic side effect of diarrhea.[10] This study provides enough data from enough studies that doctors can feel confident prescribing probiotics and patients can feel more confident and a lot better physically, too, for taking the beneficial microbes.

Probiotics don't just reduce antibiotic-associated diarrhea, they also strengthen our immune systems and gastrointestinal tract to reduce the incidence and severity of drug reactions, according to research published in the *World Journal of Gastroenterology*. The scientists found that the probiotics helped prevent adverse drug effects, modulated the immune system response, protected the gastrointestinal tract, and also promoted health.[11] Considering our goal is to boost our immunity (and not suffering) and experience health, that's great news from the scientific community.

When we also consider that many antibiotics are waning in effectiveness, taking probiotics alongside them is a double-pronged attack on harmful infectious diseases. If the antibiotics are ineffective against the bacterial intruders in our body, the probiotics are the second line of defense against them (or perhaps first in the case of resistant drugs). It may not guarantee that the intruders are destroyed, but a growing amount of research suggests that it may help to overcome them. You'll learn more about the specific probiotic superheroes against colds, flu, and superbugs in chapter 4.

An imbalance in gut microbes can further allow harmful bacteria and yeasts to multiply, which can result in additional symptoms, depending on the type of infections present. Dysbiosis can increase permeability of the intestinal walls, making it easier for harmful microbes to hijack the nutrient-shuttling system used by the body for nutrient absorption into the bloodstream. When this happens, intestinal waste products and harmful microbes gain direct access to the bloodstream, which is also known as a leaky gut or leaky gut syndrome. While this condition isn't currently well-accepted in the medical world (although I was impressed to see that Harvard University discussed this topic on its website), a more porous gut may play a role in autoimmune conditions like celiac disease, lupus, multiple sclerosis, and rheumatoid arthritis. Additional research may help to shed a light on the role of increased gut permeability and its possible connection to autoimmune conditions.

Antibiotic use isn't the only factor for gut microbial imbalances or other gut health issues, but it is certainly one of the main ones. We'll explore other issues, along with the ways to address them, throughout *Super-Powered Immunity Starts in the Gut,* but let's begin by assessing whether you might have what is known as dysbiosis—an imbalance of harmful microbes to beneficial ones.

Is Your Gut Microbiome Imbalanced?

There are many symptoms and conditions that are often linked to an imbalance of harmful to beneficial microorganisms within the intestines.[12,13] The list below is not a complete list, but some of the most common ones. Please keep in mind that this quiz is an assessment tool that is intended for educational purposes only and should not replace a physician's assessment, diagnosis, or testing. It's also important to realize that these symptoms/conditions can be linked to other health issues, so you should always consult a physician to rule out other possible health issues.

Give yourself one point for each symptom or condition you have experienced within the last few months, except where stated otherwise.

- abdominal pain or cramping
- acne
- allergies
- anxiety
- any physician-diagnosed disorder of the digestive tract (colitis, Crohn's disease, etc.). Even if you have multiple physician-diagnosed gastrointestinal (GI) disorders, count as one. (score 3)
- autoimmune disorders (rheumatoid arthritis, lupus, Hashimoto's thyroiditis, etc.) (score 3)
- bad breath
- bloating
- brain fog
- brittle hair or nails
- burping
- chronic fatigue syndrome diagnosed by a doctor (score 3)

- coated tongue (white coating that appears on the surface of the tongue)
- constipation (fewer than two healthy bowel movements daily, straining to use the bathroom, or having small, unformed stools)
- diarrhea
- eczema or psoriasis
- fibromyalgia (score 3)
- flatulence
- heartburn
- indigestion
- liver dysfunction
- sluggish lymphatic system
- stomach or duodenal ulcers
- yeast infections (oral, intestinal, or vaginal) (score 3)

0–8: If you scored 0–8, you may have a mild microbial imbalance worth addressing using the strategies you'll discover in this book.

9–18: If you scored 9–18, it is likely that you would benefit from boosting beneficial microbes in your gastrointestinal tract.

19–44: If you scored 19–44, it is likely that you are suffering from a gut microbial imbalance and should consider following the dietary and lifestyle strategies discussed in this book along with some of the remedies for killing harmful microbes.

YOU ARE WHAT YOU EAT

As you've learned, the foods and the nutrients they contain become the cells, tissues, and organs of your body, which means you literally are what you eat. Unfortunately, if the foods you choose are more junk food than nutritious, then you'll likely find yourself more vulnerable to disease. That's in part because your body attempts to make new cells from inadequate nutrition. But poor food choices can impact your gut and immune health in other ways as well. Let's explore these choices and their impact.

The Not-So-Sweet Impact of Sugar

Sugar is not only one of the most addictive substances to which we're exposed, it is also one of the most damaging to our gut and immune system health. Perhaps it wouldn't be as harmful if we weren't eating it to the tune of 152 pounds per person per year, whereas the average person ate about two pounds of sugar per year two hundred years ago.[14] Shockingly, we eat that much in under one week.

Part of the reason we eat so much sugar is that it is nearly ubiquitous in our food supply. You probably already know that it is present in high amounts in most processed, packaged, and prepared foods, but it is also found in many unexpected places. According to Nancy Appleton's classic book on the topic, *Lick the Sugar Habit*, here are some of sugar's surprising hiding places:

- The breading on most packaged and restaurant foods contains sugar.
- Sugar (in the form of corn syrup and dehydrated molasses) is often added to hamburgers sold in restaurants to reduce meat shrinkage during cooking.
- Before salmon is canned, it is often glazed with a sugar solution.
- Many meat packers feed sugar to animals prior to slaughter to "improve" flavor and color of cured meat.
- Some fast-food restaurants sell poultry that has been injected with a sugar or honey solution.
- Some salt contains sugar! Seriously.

- Sugar is used in the processing of luncheon meats, bacon, and canned meats.
- Most bouillon cubes contain sugar (and usually MSG as well).
- Peanut butter tends to contain sugar.
- Dry cereals often contain high amounts of sugar.
- Almost half of the calories from commercial ketchup comes from sugar.
- More than 90 percent of the calories found in a can of cranberry sauce come from sugar.

This doesn't include naturally occurring sugars found in fruit, vegetables, grains, and legumes. All of the above refers to added sugar only.

Remember, we are not talking about naturally occurring sugars in fruit, vegetables, grains, and legumes. We get more than enough sugar in our diets by eating these foods without adding additional sugars through processing or preparation. Industrial sugar processing has brought this sweet killer to more and more people over the last century, increasing a host of diseases and disorders that have reached epidemic proportions.

We're well aware of the connection between sugar consumption and weight gain, but few people realize that it also throws off the delicate microbial balance in the gut. That's because added sugar feeds many harmful microbes including infectious bacteria and candida yeasts, which we'll discuss in greater detail momentarily. Additionally, ingesting even a small amount of sugar can reduce our immune system function for several hours, making us more vulnerable to infections during that time. Consider how many people come down with a cold or flu during the holiday season. It may be easy to blame those with whom we've come in contact, but our higher sugar consumption also plays a role.

Reducing sugar intake is the first place to begin to restore gut health. Eating fewer processed, prepared, and packaged foods is an integral part of reducing sugar intake. It is also important to read ingredients labels on any packaged foods you select. While they won't always be listed, you'll likely find sugar or high-fructose corn syrup somewhere on the list. Additionally, sugar has many names, most of which end in the letters "ose," like fructose, lactose, maltose, and dextrose. If you see ingredients ending in "-ose" you can bet there is added sugar in the foods you're purchasing and these foods are best avoided or greatly reduced when you want to boost your gut health and immunity to disease.

While it may be tempting to assume that high-fructose corn syrup is a healthier option since it is derived from a vegetable, it is not. The average American currently consumes fifty-five pounds of high-fructose corn syrup every year, which is higher per capita consumption than any other country. Not only is elevated high-fructose corn syrup consumption linked to higher type 2 diabetes rates,[15] a study published in *Clinical and Translational Immunology* found that it can lead to inflammation in immune system cells, causing them to overreact to foreign substances and increasing the cytokine response.[16] As you may recall from our earlier discussion, the cytokine response can be valuable, but if it overreacts, it can have disastrous consequences when dealing with infectious diseases. It is unclear why high-fructose corn syrup has this effect on the immune system, but researchers believe it reprograms them.

High-fructose corn syrup also contributes to serious problems in the gut. Previously believed to be metabolized in the liver, research published in the journal *Cell Metabolism* found that high-fructose corn syrup is also metabolized in the small intestines, where it causes a deterioration of the integrity of the small intestine walls[17]—a key component of the gut-associated lymphoid tissue (GALT) that we discussed in chapter 1.

In an animal study published in the online journal *PLOS One,* researchers found that high-fructose corn syrup consumption induced an imbalance in gut microbes—dysbiosis—reducing the richness, balance, and diversity of microbes in the intestines.[18]

As more and more research shows, high-fructose corn syrup consumption, through the ingestion of fast foods, prepared foods, condiments, and other foods that contain this toxic ingredient, is impairing the gut and immune system and may be putting us at risk of serious health issues.

What Happens in Your Gut when You Eat a Low-Carb Diet?

While it's a good idea to reduce the amount of added sugar in your diet, it may be tempting to select a low-carb or high-protein dietary option. Many people select this type of diet as a way to lose weight without any consideration as to the long-term effects on their health, and certainly without consideration of the effects on the gut and immune system.

According to a study published in *Applied and Environmental Microbiology,* which explored the effects of a low-carb diet on the gut microbiome, this approach to eating may have consequences on our microbiome. Scientists at the Department of Biochemistry and Molecular Biology at Wright State University in Dayton, Ohio, used a "human gut simulator" to assess the effects of two different types of diet on the gut.[19]

The study found that a high-fat, low-carb diet increased strains of bacteria that break down fats. The switch from a balanced diet to a ketogenic-type diet caused a reduction in whole bacterial groups, including: *Bacteroides, Clostridium,* and *Roseburia,* all of which assist in the breakdown of protein and carb foods. The reduction in these bacteria produced a reduction in fatty acids and antioxidants—compounds that are needed to heal damage to DNA, as well as fight aging, inflammation, and diseases.

Bacterial diversity in the intestines is important to our overall health. And diet goes a long way toward ensuring the health of our microbiome. An earlier study published in the medical journal *Nature* showed that diet rapidly alters the microorganisms residing in our gut. The Harvard-based research found that what we eat can have drastic effects on both the numbers of microbes as well as the diversity of strains found in the intestines.[20]

Additionally, the study showed that the microbiome can shift quickly in response to diet—in as little as 24 hours after eating a meal of large quantities of animal protein, scientists found that the microbes found in the food (bacteria, fungi, and viruses) quickly colonized the gut. And, perhaps most notably, they discovered that an animal-based diet (high protein, high fat, low carb) caused the growth of microorganisms that are capable of triggering inflammatory bowel disease within only two days of eating these foods.

It is worth noting that the study was a small-scale study that explored dietary extremes by getting participants to eat a breakfast of eggs and bacon, a lunch of ribs and briskets, and salami, prosciutto, and assorted cheeses for dinner, along with pork rinds for snacks. Obviously, few people eat this way, so it is unlikely to have the same effect in people who eat more moderate amounts of meat, but the researchers wanted to get a clear picture of the effects of excessive amounts of these foods. Then, the participants switched diets and ate a plant-based diet of granola for breakfast, jasmine rice, cooked onions, tomatoes, squash, garlic, peas, and lentils for lunch, and a similar dinner, with bananas and mangoes for snacks.

In another study researchers fed rats a diet of salami, chocolate, chips, and biscuits—or what they called the "cafeteria diet." As part of an obesity study published in the journal *Age,* researchers gave some of the rats probiotics while others did not receive the beneficial bacteria. Scientists found that the probiotics were effective in preventing obesity because they had an anti-inflammatory effect on the gut and the body.[21]

While this type of research is still in its infancy, and indeed our understanding of the human microbiome is also in the early stages, it is clear that diet produces a quick and profound effect on our gut and the microbes found in it. That's not surprising when you consider a basic fact: beneficial microbes, or probiotics, are like all living beings: they need food to survive. Known as *pre*biotics, which is essentially the food for these beneficial bacteria, they are primarily found in the form of naturally occurring sugars and fiber found in plant-based foods. Knowing that, it isn't really surprising that when we eat more of these primarily carbohydrate-type plant foods, we should expect to see the numbers of beneficial microbes increase in our gut. Great health truly does begin in the gut.

Does that mean you need to go vegan and eliminate all meat, poultry, eggs, fish, and dairy from your diet? No, of course not. It simply means becoming more aware of how your food choices impact your microbiome and increasing beneficial foods that support its health. It isn't necessary to deprive yourself of your favorite foods but to simply add more vegetables, legumes, nuts, and seeds replete with nutrients, fiber, and even some natural sugars, like those found in fruit, in moderation.

A Salty Impact on Your Gut Health

Before you grab that salt shaker, keep reading. There's more reason than ever to reduce your sodium intake. In addition to the well-established link between high-salt diets and heart issues, new research found that a high-salt diet can have other harmful effects, including on your gut health.

Research published in the journal *Nature* found that a high-salt diet—the Standard American Diet (SAD) constitutes a high-salt diet—destroyed beneficial bacteria in the gut.[22,23] Researchers found that a high-sodium diet and its harmful impact on the gut may actually be one of the reasons why so many health conditions like high blood pressure and autoimmune conditions may be worsened by high-sodium diets. Conversely the scientists believe that probiotic supplementation may help to reverse some of these dietary-linked health problems, which is great news for people suffering from many different health conditions.

While experts differ on the amount of sodium needed in the diet, the American Heart Association (AHA) estimates that the average American eats more than twice as much salt as they should be. The average person ingests approximately 3,400 milligrams daily while the recommended limit is 1,500 milligrams daily.[24] A single fast-food meal in a day typically surpasses the daily limit without any other meals or snacks in a day. For example, a McDonald's quarter pounder with bacon and cheese contains around 1,380 milligrams of sodium, and that's not including the french fries or soda that typically accompany it, which push the amount to well over the maximum daily limit. So, when you consider the dietary habits of the average person, it's fair to assume that she or he probably lacks the beneficial bacteria needed for good health.

Fortunately, it is easy to cut down on salt:

- Opt for homemade meals over fast food or packaged foods.
- Make your own sauces, condiments, and salad dressings since these packaged foods tend to be extremely high in salt. Use them sparingly if you must use them.
- Choose fresh or dried herbs or herbal blends instead of salt to season your food.
- Add a splash of vinegar or lemon juice to homemade soups, salad dressings, or other foods instead of salt.
- Make your own seasoning mixes since most packaged ones tend to be high in salt.
- Start reading nutrition labels on the packaged foods you purchase and stay away from those that are high in sodium.

GIVE YOUR GUT A MICROBIAL BOOST

It's easy to give your gut a microbial boost. Here are a few of my preferred ways (and I'll share many more in chapter 6):

- Eat probiotic-rich fermented foods like sauerkraut (from the refrigerator section of your grocery or health food store), kimchi, vegan yogurt, or other foods with live cultures.
- Eat more plant-based foods since the natural fiber in these foods acts as food for beneficial bacteria and gives them a boost in your gut.

- Eat less sugar. Harmful bacteria and yeasts feed on sugar and cause the balance of good to harmful bacteria to shift in favor of the latter.
- Eat more fiber-rich foods like legumes, seeds, nuts, and whole grains. The fiber feeds beneficial microbes.

It's easier than you think to improve your gut health. Simple changes made on a daily basis can have a transformative effect on your microbiome, which in turn can have a profound impact on your immunity and overall health.

3

Probiotic-Powered Immunity

Meet the Family

In "Probiotic-Powered Immunity: Meet the Family," you'll learn the little-known secrets of probiotics that go well beyond popping a daily pill. You'll discover:

- some of the most common strains of beneficial bacteria and their main functions;
- the main families of probiotics and the parts of your gut they colonize;
- how they work to keep you healthy and ensure your survival;
- some beneficial yeasts that you'll want to obtain in your diet; and
- more essential information about probiotics.

Now that you know how important probiotic bacteria and yeasts are to your health and life, let's meet the microorganisms that share your journey through life with you. The two main types of bacteria are known as Lactobacilli and Bifidobacteria. Each of these groups of bacteria has many species and subspecies performing critical functions in your body, including: the formation and absorption of essential nutrients, detoxifying toxic substances, stimulating the immune system against harmful bacteria and viruses, and preventing gut inflammation and disease elsewhere in your body, to name a few.

Some of these many healing probiotics include: the Lactobacilli family. Lactobacillus is usually shortened to L. when listing them. This family includes: *L. acidophilus, L. brevis, L. bulgaricus, L. casei, L. gasseri, L. paracasei, L. plantarum,* and others. The Bifidobacteria family, which are usually shortened to B. when listing them, include: *B. bifidum, B. breve, B. infantis, B. lactis,* and others. There are other beneficial bacteria like *Streptococcus thermophilus*; as well as beneficial yeasts and fungi (such as *Saccharomyces boulardii*).

Let's meet the families that are helping you maintain strong health and immunity every second of every day.

THE LACTOBACILLI FAMILY

The Lactobacilli family includes the most commonly known strains of probiotics. They are largely found in the small intestines, as well as the genitals, mouth, nose, throat, and upper respiratory tract. They are involved in a wide range of functions including cellular renewal to keep the intestinal walls healthy and intact. If you're suffering from intestinal issues, you may benefit from increased Lactobacilli.

Pregnant women tend to have large colonies of Lactobacilli, which inoculate a newborn baby during the birth process so she or he will have the necessary microbes for a healthy life.

Some of the many strains of Lactobacilli include: *L. acidophilus, L. brevis, L. bulgaricus, L. casei, L. delbrueckii, L. gasseri, L. johnsonii, L. paracasei, L. plantarum, L. reuteri, L. rhamnosus,* and *L. salivarius.* While each strain performs unique functions, they all produce lactic acid and hydrogen peroxide in the intestines, both of which have natural antimicrobial properties that can help kill harmful bacteria, fungi, and viruses. They also trigger proteins produced by the white blood cells that have an anti-inflammatory effect and respond to harmful infectious invaders of our body.

During food fermentation processes, Lactobacilli convert sugars to lactic acid, making them valuable both from a health perspective but also for food preservation. This is the process used to ferment foods like pickles (not quick pickles, but naturally fermented ones), sauerkraut, and yogurt. Other fermented foods, which we'll discuss in chapter 5, including kombucha (fermented tea), sourdough bread, and vinegar, among others, ferment as a result of Lactobacilli.

Lactobacillus acidophilus—The Pioneer

The first discovered probiotic is also one of the most valuable. Found in yogurt with live cultures, it helps the fermentation of milk sugars, as well as other sugars and carbohydrates (starches). It has even been found to reduce the symptoms of lactose intolerance by improving the metabolism of milk sugar, known as lactose, during digestion and in transit through the GI tract. As a result, it may be valuable for digestion in general. It is important to replenish these probiotics after a course of antibiotics.[1]

Lactobacillus brevis—The Anticancer Booster

Because *L. brevis* adheres well to the walls of the intestines, it helps to crowd out less desirable, disease-causing microbes, preventing them from adhering, which they need to do for their survival. According to a study in the journal *Anticancer Research,* scientists have identified *L. brevis* as potentially having anticancer effects.[2]

Lactobacillus bulgaricus—The Antimicrobial Cholesterol Reducer

A close relative of *L. acidophilus, L. bulgaricus* is widely used in the production of cheeses and yogurt. In a study published in the journal *Frontiers in Microbiology,* scientists found that this probiotic demonstrated antimicrobial effects against harmful bacteria and helped to restore normal cholesterol levels. Like its Lactobacilli counterparts, it also reduces inflammation, which is a factor in most health conditions.[3]

Lactobacillus casei—The Lactose Alleviator

L. casei helps to digest milk sugars known as lactose and may even help to alleviate lactose intolerance. It also reduces cholesterol levels, enhances immune response, inhibits intestinal pathogens, and controls diarrhea, making this probiotic a potentially good option for a wide variety of health issues.[4]

Lactobacillus gasseri—The Bacteria Destroyer

L. gasseri produces compounds called bacteriocins that may be helpful in the destruction of harmful bacteria.[5] It has also been linked to breaking down compounds known as urinary oxalates, which are linked to kidney stones,[6] which may make this probiotic beneficial for the treatment of kidney stones, as well as infectious bacterial conditions.

Lactobacillus plantarum—The Gut Restorer

If you eat the Standard American Diet, there's a chance you may lack the probiotic known as *L. plantarum,* which as the name might suggest is typically found in plants and therefore those who eat them. It is known for regulating the immune system and as a possible treatment for those suffering from irritable bowel syndrome (IBS) and irritable bowel disease (IBD).[7]

Lactobacillus reuteri—The Antimicrobial Magician

L. reuteri is a versatile probiotic that is involved in many functions that help preserve and restore health, including the production of a compound called reuterin, an antimicrobial compound that inhibits the growth of harmful bacteria, fungi, and other microbes. As a result, it is believed to hold promise as a therapy to alleviate certain conditions linked to the gastrointestinal system, oral health, urinary tract and genital health, as well as eczema and *H. pylori* infections,[8] the latter of which have been linked to ulcers.

Lactobacillus rhamnosus—The Great Gut Warrior

While it may sound more like the name of an Egyptian god, *L. rhamnosus* is a warrior against harmful microbes thanks to its ability to adhere to cells, colonize the intestines, and crowd or destroy harmful microbes through their own ability to proliferate.[9] As a result, it likely holds great promise in the treatment of a wide variety of gastrointestinal and other health issues.

Lactobacillus salivarius—The Bacteria Slayer

Another anti-microbial powerhouse probiotic, due to its ability to produce compounds known as bacteriocins that kill harmful bacteria, *L. salivarius* holds promise in the treatment of serious infectious conditions including the antibiotic-resistant bacterial infection known as *Staphylococcus aureus*. It appears to have the ability to break down biofilms created by the infectious bacteria, better enabling the body to fight. Additionally, *L. salivarius* shows antimicrobial activity against *E. coli, Salmonella,* and *Listeria,* making it an excellent choice in the potential treatment of harmful bacteria.

Are Harmful Bacteria Resistant to Probiotics?

Antibiotic resistance can be deadly when it comes to harmful bacteria that cause infectious disease, but it is worth noting that some beneficial microbes (probiotics) have also developed resistance to antibiotic drugs. In other words, even broad-spectrum antibiotic drugs cannot kill some of these beneficial microbes. However, antibiotic-resistant probiotics are actually beneficial for our health, particularly for people taking antibiotic drugs along with probiotic supplements. In such a situation, the antibiotics that normally indiscriminately kill bacteria may actually leave some probiotics intact where they can continue to populate your intestines.

Scientists at four Chinese universities collaborated to assess one hundred strains of probiotic bacteria to determine whether they had become antibiotic resistant. They conducted tests on many strains and substrains of probiotic bacteria. They found that all of the probiotics tested were resistant to the antibiotics gentamicin and streptomycin; forty-two were resistant to the drug vancomycin; and all had some degree of sensitivity to the antibiotics cephalexin, erythromycin, tetracycline, and oxytetracycline.[10]

So how does that unfold in the real world, and what does it mean to you? It means that you'll still want to replenish probiotics if you're taking a course of antibiotic drugs; however, it may also mean that over time antibiotics may have less potency against beneficial microbes. So, you may also experience fewer gut disturbances, such as antibiotic-induced diarrhea, from taking antibiotics. But, the truth is, we don't really know for sure where this is going as we haven't been here before. It's all new, so while you wait for the researchers to sort things out, you may want to keep taking your probiotic supplements, particularly if you're also taking antibiotics, and you'll want to incorporate a wide range of delicious fermented foods into your daily life. Don't like one variety of kimchi, yogurt, or sauerkraut? Keep trying different ones until you find options you love.

THE BIFIDOBACTERIA FAMILY

While the Lactobacilli family gets most of the credit for the therapeutic benefits of probiotics and fermented foods, they aren't the only beneficial microbes helping to keep us healthy. The Bifidobacteria family of beneficial bacteria are commonly found in the gastrointestinal tract, mouth, and vagina. Their function varies from strain to strain, but they collectively confer the benefits of the creation of anticancer compounds, vitamin production, destroying infection-causing microbes, and helping to balance the immune system.[11]

There are about seven times as many Bifidobacteria as there are Lactobacilli in a healthy adult human gut. They tend to be strong immune boosters and are usually found in fermented vegetables, kefir, kombucha, sauerkraut, and yogurt. Don't worry if you're not familiar with all of these fermented foods, as we'll discuss them in greater detail in chapter 5.

There are approximately thirty *Bifidobacterium* strains identified to date, and you'll often see them shortened to B. when mentioned in texts or identified on ingredient labels of products. Some of the most common ones include: *B. bifidum, B. breve, B. infantis, B. lactis,* and *B. longum.* Let's explore these five beneficial Bifidobacteria.

Bifidobacterium bifidum—The Bowel Balancer

In a study published in the journal *Lancet Gastroenterology and Hepatology,* researchers found that *Bifidobacterium bifidum,* or *B. bifidum* as it is also known, significantly alleviated irritable bowel syndrome (IBS) and its symptoms,[12] some of which include: abdominal pain, bloating, cramping, diarrhea or constipation (or alternating between the two), and gas.[13]

Bifidobacterium breve—The Infection Eliminator

When it comes to fighting infectious microbes, *Bifidobacterium breve* is quickly demonstrating its prowess. These beneficial bacteria secrete enzymes that alter the intestinal microbes, killing harmful ones linked to infections and diseases, including *C. difficile* and a group called *Bacteroides.* While the latter can be beneficial in the intestines, when their numbers become high or they migrate outside of the intestines, they can be responsible for harmful infections and abscesses.[14]

B. breve is also demonstrating potency against *Campylobacter jejuni*[15] and rotavirus.[16]

Bifidobacterium infantis—The Baby Gut Booster

You can probably guess from the scientific name of this bacterium where it is typically found: the intestines of infants. It is a naturally anti-inflammatory probiotic that is actually a subspecies of *Bifidobacterium longum,* found in infants. It has the ability to reduce inflammatory processes in the gut and beyond. It also helps to regulate the immune system and plays an important role in the gut of infants and children.[17]

Bifidobacterium lactis—The Immune Supercharger

Bifidobacterium lactis is also known as *Bifidobacterium animalis* (subspecies *lactis*) and is a heavily researched probiotic that demonstrates its potency against harmful microbes and its ability to enhance the gastrointestinal and immune systems. It has been shown to improve bowel functions and reduce the effect of antibiotics, including reducing the incidence of antibiotic-associated diarrhea. It has also been found in studies to increase the body's resistance to respiratory infections.[18]

Bifidobacterium longum—The Gut Protector

B. longum is a powerful gut healer that has been found to help reduce intestinal inflammation. It has even demonstrated effectiveness in the treatment of inflammatory bowel diseases like ulcerative colitis and Crohn's disease. Inflammatory bowel disease (IBD) is associated with changes in gut microbes and the immune system, and, as the name suggests, inflammation. This is good news for sufferers of these challenging conditions.[19] It's also good news for everyone who wants a healthy gut and immune system because this probiotic has also been found to restore microbial balance in the gut, eliminating harmful varieties and increasing beneficial ones.[20]

MORE BACTERIA WITH BENEFITS

While Lactobacilli and Bifidobacteria are the most common beneficial bacteria, they are not the only ones.

Streptococcus salivarius—The Antibacteria Bacteria

It may be surprising to learn that some strep bacteria fight other strep bacteria, but it's true. The probiotic known as *Streptococcus salivarius* has been shown in studies to secrete antibacterial compounds known as salivaricin A2 and B, both of which strongly fight another strain of strep bacteria linked to throat infections.[21] While it is most often considered a probiotic, more research needs to be done on this strain since it has been linked to cases of the blood infection known as sepsis in immunocompromised individuals. I've included it not because I think you should supplement with it, but because some supplements include it and I think it's important to be informed.[22]

Streptococcus thermophilus—The Protector

It may be tempting to cast these bacteria aside at first glance at the scientific name. While it may sound dauntingly similar to strep infections, these particular bacteria confer benefits rather than nasty health infectious conditions. Commonly used in yogurt- and cheese-making, *Streptococcus thermophilus,* or *S. thermophilus* as it is also known, can help boost the body's energy production, known as adenosine triphosphate, or ATP.[23] In an animal study, it demonstrated effectiveness against candida infections.[24] According to a study published in the journal *Gastroenterology,* it has even been shown to help protect the body against tumors in the colon.[25]

USEFUL YEASTS

We typically associate yeasts with harmful infections, and indeed, some strains are connected with illnesses like yeast infections, but there are some beneficial yeasts too. These beneficial yeasts, such as a type known as *Saccharomyces boulardii,* are not related to disease-causing ones like *Candida albicans,* for example.

Saccharomyces boulardii—The Gut Balancer

Named after the French microbiologist Henri Boulard who observed that Indo-Chinese people treated cholera-linked diarrhea with a fermented lychee and mangosteen tea. Upon examination, he found that the beverage contained a yeast strain that had not previously been identified, so he gave it the name *S. boulardii*. He patented the probiotic as an anti-diarrhea medication since *S. boulardii* is so effective against microbes that are linked with diarrhea, including *C. difficile, E. coli, Candida albicans,* and others.[26] The yeast has been found to combat a wide range of gastrointestinal disorders and has even been found effective at inhibiting cholera.[27]

Saccharomyces cerevisiae—The Fermenter

This largely probiotic yeast is often found on the skins of certain fruits and vegetables, including apples and grapes. Most notably known for its use in fermentation of wine, beer, and as a leavening agent in bread, *S. cerevisiae* can also offer beneficial therapeutic effects in some cases. In a study published in the journal *Virulence,* researchers found it exerted a beneficial effect on treating vaginal candida infections. While it is normally probiotic in nature, offering a range of beneficial effects, it may be best avoided among immunocompromised individuals.[28]

4

The Pro-Powered Superheroes against Colds, Flu, and Superbugs

In chapter 4, you'll discover:

- the potential heroes of the war against superbugs;
- an army of superheroes—probiotics—that is rising to take the place of antibiotics;
- the exciting, potentially life-saving research about particular probiotic strains that are demonstrating effectiveness against even the most drug-resistant health conditions like MRSA and *C. difficile;*
- the bacteria that fight disease-causing viruses;
- the probiotics that fight fungal infections like candida; and
- the effectiveness of probiotics against a range of other infections.

PRO-POWERED WARRIORS AGAINST VIRUSES

Can you imagine a world where at the first sign of a serious and deadly threat, a large group of warriors came to the rescue? We know that our immune systems do this. But what if our immune systems had warrior helpers that not only boosted the strength of our body's own immunity, but actually waged war on the viruses threatening our health with serious disease? You might be surprised to learn that bacteria inside your body actually perform this vital and noble function. The idea that bacteria target, wage war against, and overpower viruses sounds like the stuff of science fiction movies or novels, but a growing body of research is finding that not only do they do that, but they may actually be among our best weapons against serious viral threats. This is an area where the research on probiotics really is beginning to shine.

Whether you're exposed to a common cold, the herpes virus that causes cold sores, or a much more serious virus like those involved in HIV infections, a growing body of research is showing that probiotics may be helpful against possibly even our worst viral threats.

Colds, Flu, and Other Viruses

We mostly just live with colds and flu, knowing that our immune system, along with some soup, vitamin C, and echinacea thrown in for good measure, will overpower these annoying viruses. Yes, we may suffer for a few days or weeks, but we know, for most of us at least, that the agony will end and we'll be feeling back to ourselves in no time.

But what if we could significantly cut our risk of contracting a cold in the first place? Research published in the *European Journal of Nutrition* found that probiotic strain *L. plantarum* as well as *L. paracasei* reduced the risk of contracting the common cold. That might not sound like a big deal, but keep in mind that I'm not aware of any drug that has ever been able to achieve this impressive feat. Drugs may help us minimize symptoms, but they don't actually reduce our risk of getting a cold.

What's more: the scientists found that these probiotics cut the duration of the common cold from 8.6 days in the placebo group to 6.2 days among study participants taking probiotics. That's nearly two and a half days in which people were not suffering simply by taking probiotics.

And, if that wasn't impressive enough, those taking the probiotics also had a reduced severity of symptoms. In other words, this study demonstrated that the probiotic supplements worked against the common cold in three ways.[1] The drugs we use for the common cold do not cut our risk of contracting a cold and do not lessen the duration of the virus. They merely suppress the symptoms.

In a New Zealand study published in the *Journal of Science and Medicine in Sport,* scientists at the University of Otago assessed the effects of probiotic supplementation in rugby players in the Rugby Union. While the sample size was small—only thirty-five—the participants were elite athletes. They received either a probiotic supplement or a placebo for four weeks. Fourteen of those taking the probiotic treatment did not contract any upper respiratory tract infections compared to six who remained free of infection in the placebo group. Additionally, those in the placebo group who contracted the infection suffered for a longer duration. Although the study size was small, considering the *European Journal of Nutrition* study, as well as the safety and possible additional benefits of supplementing with probiotics, the results warrant consideration.[2]

Additional research demonstrates a similar ability of probiotics to prevent some infectious conditions and speed their healing. Scientists assessed the ability of probiotics to prevent and treat ear infections as well as respiratory infections in the *Journal of Applied Microbiology.* Their results give us fascinating insights into the wondrous microbial worlds inside our body. They discovered that probiotics compete with harmful, disease-causing microbes for space, nutrients, and even the ability to attach to human hosts. Whether or not we get sick might be determined by whether the beneficial microbes win their war against viruses that cause infections, at least in the case of the ear and respiratory infections explored in the study. The scientists found that probiotics thrive at the expense of infectious microbes, such as the viruses causing ear and respiratory infections, resulting in the disease-causing viruses to die while reducing our symptoms and illness as a side effect of their battle.[3] Now that's a side effect we can all be happy to experience.

Their potency against viruses is not the only reason to incorporate probiotics into the treatment of respiratory and ear infections. They also have a proven safety record and are safe for most people to use.

A Finnish study conducted by the Department of Pediatrics and Adolescent Medicine at University of Turku Hospital and published in the *Journal of Allergy and Clinical Immunology* found that pre-term infants suffered from fewer viral respiratory infections when they were given probiotic supplements. Ninety-four infants were given probiotics that included *L. rhamnosus* between days three to sixty of their life. The researchers concluded that the probiotic-treated infants had significantly fewer infections, indicating "probiotics might offer a novel and cost-effective means to reduce the risk of rhinovirus infections."[4] And the additional benefit was that the researchers were able to improve the health of the infants without invasive drugs or other measures.

Of course, when using probiotics with children or infants it's important to remember that not all strains of probiotics have been tested on infants and children, so stick with a product or products that are designed with them in mind for the greatest benefit and least risk. For those who are immunocompromised, you may wish to stick with the beneficial bacteria, rather than the probiotic yeasts, and consult with your physician.

The elderly may also benefit from probiotics to boost their ability to prevent or address respiratory infections. According to a French study of over a thousand elderly patients to see if yogurt containing *Lactobacillus casei* would impact the frequency with which they contracted lung infections or the duration they suffered from them, research published in the *British Journal of Nutrition* found that the probiotic-containing yogurt reduced both the frequency of upper respiratory tract infections and the amount of time the study participants suffered from infections, reducing the duration by 1.5 days compared to the placebo group.[5]

Cold Sores, Chicken Pox, and Quelling the Herpes Virus

If you've suffered from a cold sore, you're already familiar with the herpes virus. There are two types of herpes: simplex and zoster. Herpes simplex can present as either cold sores or genital herpes[6] while herpes zoster is the virus linked to chickenpox and shingles. Once we have come in contact with the herpes virus, it remains in our body, but it can return to a dormant state, which is where probiotics may be helpful.

According to Italian research published in the medical journal *Anaerobe,* the probiotic *Lactobacillus brevis* may be helpful against the herpes simplex virus. Scientists found that *L. brevis* demonstrated antiviral activity against the herpes simplex virus by inhibiting the virus's ability to multiply. The results were dose dependent, meaning that higher doses of this probiotic produced greater antiviral effects.[7] While the probiotic may be effective against herpes zoster, it simply was not assessed in this study. Additional research found that the probiotic *L. plantarum* also inhibited the herpes simplex virus.[8]

Human Immunodeficiency Virus (HIV) and Our Understanding of How Probiotics Work

We know that probiotics can be helpful in the prevention or treatment of respiratory infections and herpes virus-related conditions, but, thanks to Ukrainian research we now know that they may also be helpful against many other types of viruses, including human immunodeficiency virus, due to some strains' ability to prevent viruses from reproducing. Viruses cannot survive without replicating themselves, which is their key to infecting people.

In an animal study, Ukrainian scientists found that the probiotics *L. plantarum, S. salivarius,* and *S. thermophilus* not only demonstrated effectiveness at killing flu viruses and genital herpes, they even inhibited the ability of the HIV virus from reproducing.[9] Viruses rely on reproduction to spread throughout the body for their survival, suggesting that these two strains of probiotics may be helpful in the treatment of flu viruses and genital herpes and even the management of HIV. That's promising news to the approximately thirty-eight million people worldwide currently living with HIV, according to Avert, an organization dedicated to global information and education about HIV.[10]

HIV infection is often initially characterized by flu-like symptoms, including fatigue, fever, headaches, joint or muscle aches, rashes, sore throats, and swollen glands. Over time, those infected with the virus typically experience additional symptoms, including: depression; diarrhea that often lasts a week or longer; extreme and unexplained fatigue; memory loss; neurological symptoms; pneumonia; prolonged swelling of the lymph glands in the armpits, groin, or neck; rapid weight loss; recurring fevers or night sweats; sores of the anus, genital area, or mouth; and red, brown, pink, or purple-colored blotches on or under the skin of the mouth, nose, or eyelid regions.

Since so many of the symptoms mimic other conditions, including some that are fairly minor like the flu, it is a good idea to get tested if you suspect you may have an HIV infection. While there is currently no known cure for HIV, identifying it at its early stages may make the treatment more effective, improve quality of life, and reduce the likelihood of unknowingly infecting others. Additionally, because people who suffer with HIV often have complications from other illnesses, it can help to be informed. In that way, these conditions can be addressed using natural treatments, including probiotics and fermented foods, to minimize the symptoms and potential health damage.

Iranian researchers at the Shiraz HIV/AIDS Research Center (SHARC), Department of Bacteriology and Virology, Shiraz University of Medical Sciences, discovered that the probiotic *L. rhamnosus* enhanced the body's ability to produce a type of immune system cells called macrophages. As you learned in chapter 1, macrophage literally means "big eat" because they are relatively large cells, by comparison to others in the body at least, that engulf harmful infectious microbes and destroy them. Think Pac-Man and you'll have a good idea as to how macrophages work. Boosting the quantity of macrophages is imperative to overcoming many infectious diseases. Published in the *Brazilian Journal of Infectious Diseases,*[11] While the research is still in its infancy, incorporating *L. rhamnosus* into an HIV treatment program may be beneficial and may help to keep the immune system strong. Because the disease is often difficult to treat and frequently treated with harsh drugs replete with plentiful side effects, including natural options like probiotics that show promise and seem only to have beneficial effects may be helpful.

Research in the *Indian Journal of Pediatrics* found that probiotics could also positively influence white blood cells, which are needed for a strong immune system. Researchers at the Department of Pediatrics and Antiretroviral Therapy (ART) Center at the S. N. Medical College in Agra, India, assessed 127 HIV-infected children, all of whom were under sixteen years old. The scientists discovered that supplementation with probiotics significantly improved white blood cells known as CD4.[12] The CD4 count is a reflection of the strength of the immune system to fight viruses and is often used as an indicator to determine the stage of HIV/AIDS as the count can significantly drop in a person suffering from the disease. The researchers found that supplementing with probiotics for six months resulted in a significant increase in the CD4 count, which suggests a stronger, healthier immune system.

Other research suggests that probiotics may also boost the body's production of immune cells known as killer T cells. Published in the journal *Clinical and Experimental Immunology,* researchers assessed the effects of two probiotics, *L. plantarum* and *L. paracasei,* on the immune system to determine their possible role in enhancing immune functions. They learned that different probiotic strains, including *L. plantarum,* may have different effects on the immune system and increased the body's means of T cells that activate the immune system while *L. paracasei* increased the number of killer T cells.[13]

While we're still in the early stages of understanding how probiotics interact with our immune systems and bodies, it's exciting to know that they may be boosting the cells that engulf harmful infectious viruses, as well as those that attack them directly. But there are additional ways that probiotics may be helpful for a healthy immune system.

For women, ensuring a healthy vaginal microbiome may also reduce the risk of infections. Research published in the medical journal *FEMS Microbiology Review* found that a microbial imbalance in the vagina may make women more vulnerable to contracting infectious diseases like HIV. Known as dysbiosis, which is characterized by an imbalance of harmful microbes to beneficial ones, it may increase the risk of disease transmission. In this study, scientists found that probiotics may help to protect women against HIV in the following ways: 1) by the direct production of antiviral compounds; 2) by blocking the adhesion and transmission of the virus; and 3) by stimulating the immune response to destroy the virus.[14] At this time, research into the impact of probiotics on HIV transmission is in its infancy, but this study demonstrates their role in ensuring a healthy vaginal microbiome. Of course, it need not be stated that probiotics will not protect a person from contracting a serious disease like HIV and should not be used as a substitute for personal accountability and protection during sexual activities.

Because HIV sufferers are also frequently at risk of contracting other infectious diseases due to their reduced immune response, many suffer from candida infections. Candida is often called a yeast infection, but it is actually a fungal infection that often inhabits the intestines but can also infect the vagina and other places in the body. Caused by any of 150 species of fungi that are collectively known as *Candida, Candida albicans* is one of the most common ones involved in candida infections, or candidiasis as it is also called. Some of the symptoms include allergies, bloating, brain fog, chemical sensitivities, chronic fatigue, depression, diarrhea or constipation, gas, irritability, reduced resistance to infections, skin conditions (acne, eczema, psoriasis, for example), PMS, thrush, and vaginal yeast infections.

Those suffering from HIV often suffer from co-infections like candida largely because their immune systems are significantly reduced. In a study published in the medical journal *Mycopathologia,* scientists analyzed the effects of probiotic-rich yogurt on candida infections. In this study, twenty-four women abstained from probiotics for sixty days, then consumed probiotic-rich yogurt for fifteen days, followed by a thirty-day "washout" period in which they, once again, did not consume probiotics. The researchers took mouth and vaginal swabs at the start of the study and once again on days sixty and seventy-four to determine whether the probiotics had any effect on the candida infections. They found less *Candida* when the women consumed probiotics (29 percent versus 54 percent in the nonprobiotic time).[15] Although the study is a small pilot study, it may be helpful in addressing co-infections linked to HIV.

Probiotics against *H. Pylori* Infections in the Gut

You may have heard of *Helicobacter pylori* (*H. pylori*) infections as there has been a growing concern about bacterial infections like this one being successfully treated with antibiotics. The infection often appears after excessive use of nonsteroidal anti-inflammatory drugs (NSAIDs), which can aggravate the GI tract and can be at the root of ulcers and gastritis.[16] Peptic ulcers involve painful sores or ulcerations in the stomach or upper intestinal tract, while gastritis involves inflammation, irritation, or erosion of the stomach lining.[17]

According to the *World Journal of Gastroenterology, H. pylori* has infected approximately 4.4 billion people worldwide.[18]

While the incidence of the infections as well as its growing resistance to antibiotics are cause for concern, the news isn't all bad: probiotics involving certain strains of bacteria have been found to slow or halt growth of *H. pylori* and may be beneficial in the treatment of these conditions.

Scientists found that probiotics work against *H. pylori* bacteria and improve general gastrointestinal health in five ways. Here are some of their exciting findings:

1. Bacteria in the Lactobacilli family reinforce the protective functions in the stomach and GI tract by maintaining bacterial balance.

2. Probiotic bacteria secrete various substances that may inhibit or destroy *H. pylori* bacteria. These substances include certain types of fats known as short-chain fatty acids (SCFAs) and bacteriocins. Bacteriocins are compounds with antibacterial activity. It may seem strange to think of probiotic bacteria as secreting antibacterial compounds, but when you consider that they are competing with other bacteria for food and space, it makes more sense.

3. Probiotic bacteria seem to prevent the ability of bacteria, including *H. pylori,* of adhering to the walls of the GI tract, thereby preventing the ability of *H. pylori* to survive.

4. *H. pylori* has been shown in studies to affect gene expression in cells of the GI tract to cause reduced mucus secretion. Conversely, research shows that *L. plantarum* and *L. rhamnosus* improve the expression of the genes involved, further inhibiting the ability of harmful bacteria like *H. pylori* to survive.

5. Probiotics show the ability to regulate the immune system's response to *H. pylori* bacteria (and others) by reducing inflammatory compounds.[19]

There is still some uncertainty as to which strains may be best, but a few seem to be standing out in this regard, including *Bifidobacteria bifiform, L. johnsonii, L. plantarum, L. reuteri, L. rhamnosus,* and *Saccharomyces boulardii.*

In one study, the probiotic *Bifidobacteria bifiform* demonstrated the ability to improve the effectiveness of the typical antibiotic treatment for *H. pylori,* reduced the drug side effects at the same time, and also boosted the body's immune system against *H. pylori.*[20]

Multiple animal studies demonstrate that probiotics reduce *H. pylori* infections as well as the resulting gut inflammation linked to the harmful bacteria.[21–25] Scientists at the University of Chile, in Santiago found an impressive number of people who took the probiotic *L. johnsonii* along with pure cranberry juice, which is often used in the treatment of *H. pylori* infections, had eradicated 22.9 percent of *H. pylori,* while the placebo group experienced an eradication rate of *H. pylori* of only 1.5 percent. Those who exclusively used the probiotic experienced a 14.9 percent eradication of *H. pylori,* which was also significantly higher than the placebo group. The combination of pure cranberry juice, not the sweetened varieties on the market, combined with the probiotic *L. johnsonii* had the greatest effectiveness against *H. pylori* infections.[26]

Other research published in the *World Journal of Gastroenterology* found that the probiotic strains *L. johnsonii, L. reuteri,* and *Saccharomyces boulardii* showed the greatest effectiveness against *H. pylori,* while *L. paracasei, L. acidophilus LB, L. rhamnosus, B. animalis,* and *L. gasseri OLL2716* have only been minimally effective or not effective at all.[27]

While the research continues to further explore effective strains against *H. pylori,* including the best doses to take, it may be beneficial to incorporate a probiotic supplement with one or more of the above strains of probiotics in it as part of your treatment plan along with my seven-step plan outlined in chapter 6 to address *H. pylori* infections.

Probiotics for Oral Health

While we don't often consider the mouth as part of the gastrointestinal tract, digestion actually begins there, through the process of chewing our food and by initiating the breakdown of carbohydrates. It's imperative that we have healthy digestion that begins in the mouth for the benefit of a strong gut and because harmful bacteria that can build up in the mouth can access the bloodstream, where they can cause further damage.

Fortunately, probiotics have shown promise in the treatment of oral and dental disorders, including periodontitis, which is a gum infection that causes inflammation, damages the soft tissue in the mouth, and can also destroy the bone that supports your teeth.[28]

While it is a common problem, sadly it also increases the risk of suffering a heart attack or stroke. As a result, it's imperative to address the condition as soon as possible. Probiotics may be beneficial in this capacity.

A study published in the *Journal of Clinical Periodontology* found that the use of probiotic lozenges containing *Lactobacillus reuteri* taken for twelve weeks resulted in a reduction in the harmful bacteria linked to the condition.[29]

Pro Power against Serious Staph Infections

We know that our perceived best antibiotic drugs are not working against some bacteria, *Staphylococcus aureus,* which has become resistant to the main antibiotic used to fight it—methicillin. You may have heard about MRSA being found in hospital settings and sadly having deadly consequences for many people. MRSA stands for methicillin-resistant *Staphylococcus aureus,* which often strikes when people are most vulnerable, such as in hospitals when they are admitted for other health issues. While the mainstream media have been extensively reporting on the seriousness of the situation and the fact that antibiotic drugs are reducing in effectiveness against the bacterial infection, I have never seen a news report showcasing the natural options like probiotics that are demonstrating effectiveness. The study of probiotics in the treatment of MRSA is still in its infancy, but it warrants attention.

In a study published in the *International Journal of Antimicrobial Agents,* researchers found that probiotics played a role in both the prevention and treatment of methicillin-resistant *Staphylococcus aureus* infections. After reviewing the literature on probiotics used against MRSA, the researchers found that many strains exhibited antibacterial activity against the superbug that causes the disease. Their study found that the most active strains include: *L. reuteri, L. rhamnosus, L. paracasei, L. acidophilus, L. casei, L. plantarum, L. bulgaricus, L. fermentum,* and *L. lactis,* as well as some little-known and likely hard-to-obtain strains.

They concluded that these probiotics worked on *S. aureus* in three ways: 1) competing with *S. aureus* bacteria for nutrients and attachment; 2) producing antibacterial compounds known as "bacteriocins" and acids that kill infectious bacteria; and 3) inhibiting the harmful bacteria from producing what is known as a "biofilm" that protects it and reduces the likelihood of being detected and killed by the immune system. By slowing or stopping *S. aureus*'s ability to form biofilms, the probiotics better enabled the immune system to fight off the harmful pathogen. The scientists concluded that the research "pointed to the feasibility of elimination or reduction of MRSA colonisation with probiotic use."[30]

Other research published in the *Journal of Medical Microbiology* found that *B. longum* and *B. animalis* (*lactis*) inhibited the growth of various strains of MRSA.[31] While there is no guarantee that these probiotic strains will be effective against all MRSA infections, it's exciting to know that probiotics may help us in dealing with these serious microbes. That's good news considering that the inappropriate use of antibiotics may eliminate the beneficial bacteria that protect the skin, making it more difficult to fight MRSA skin infections.[32] As we increasingly rely on antibacterial hand sanitizers to indiscriminately kill all microbes on our hands, the potential use of probiotics to help us battle MRSA could not be timelier.

Naturally Tackling *C. Diff* Infections

Probiotics may be helpful for tackling other superbugs like *C. difficile* infections. Research published in the *International Journal of Infectious Diseases* found that probiotics are demonstrating effectiveness for the prevention and treatment of *C. difficile*. This is important since the researchers indicated that *C. diff* infections have "surpassed methicillin-resistant *Staphylococcus aureus* as the number one cause of hospital-acquired infections in some areas of the USA."[33]

Research published in the journal *Current Opinion in Gastroenterology* found that probiotic use may reduce the incidence of

C. difficile infections by 50 percent.[34] Additional research published in the journal *Clinical Infectious Diseases* had similar results, yielding a marked reduction in the incidence of *C. diff* infections using supplementation with *L. acidophilus, L. casei,* and *L. rhamnosus.*[35] While the scientists obtained results with these three probiotics, there may be others that work as well, but they were not assessed in this study.

Probiotics Assist with Fungal Infections

It's incredible to think of bacteria doing battle with fungi, but that's exactly what happens in your body when it comes to fungal infections like candidiasis, which is caused by any number of fungal strains collectively known as *Candida.* Probiotic supplementation (and of course regular consumption of fermented foods) is essential to controlling the fungal overgrowth, regardless of whether they exist in the gut, mouth, or vagina.

Most women suffer from vaginal yeast infections at some point in their lifetime; many deal with them on a frequent basis. Sadly, antibiotics are often prescribed to treat these infections, which indiscriminately kill the beneficial bacteria needed in the vagina to fight the infections. You may recall our earlier discussion that antibiotics work on bacteria, not fungi, and therefore will not yield the desired outcome when used to treat candida.

There are oral probiotic products on the market that can be used in the prevention and treatment of oral, gut, or vaginal candida infections, as well as probiotic vaginal suppositories that can be used in the treatment of vaginal infections. Research at the Lawson Health Research Institute, Canadian Research and Development Center for Probiotics found that a combination of two probiotic strains, *L. rhamnosus* and *L. fermentum,* taken orally resulted in a significant increase in vaginal Lactobacilli at days 28 and 60 of their study—the days they conducted their assessments. The researchers also identified a sharp decline in yeast at day 28 and a significant reduction in coliform bacteria (such as *E. coli*), which are also involved in vaginal infections, at days 28, 60, and 90 for the Lactobacilli-treated women. Thirty-seven percent of women taking the probiotic supplement who had vaginal bacterial or yeast infections returned to normal microbe colonization while only 13 percent of the placebo group not taking the probiotics experienced a return to normal, healthy microbial colonies. Scientists concluded that this probiotic combination reduces the colonization of pathogenic bacteria and yeast in the vagina and is safe for daily use in healthy women.[36]

Of course, the study explored probiotics exclusively, not in combination with herbal antimicrobials and dietary and lifestyle changes, all of which would likely increase the number of women who overcome the harmful vaginal infections. You'll learn my multifaceted plan, along with some of the best remedies against *Candida* and other harmful gut infections, in chapter 6.

Causes of Candida Infection

Antibiotic use and a high-sugar, high-meat, high-salt diet, among other factors, can cause serious imbalances in the gut, creating an intestinal environment where other harmful microbes can thrive.

There are many types of opportunistic infections that can inhabit our intestines, but one of the most common is known as *Candida albicans*. Candida, as it is often called, is usually referred to as a yeast infection, but it is actually a type of fungus. While we often think of women as being vulnerable to these infections, as this fungus also contributes to vaginal infections, men and women alike suffer from candida infections of the GI tract. There are many species of fungi that are collectively known as *Candida*, but *Candida albicans* is one of the most common.

There are many causes of candida infections, however, some of the most common ones include:

alcohol consumption;

chlorinated water;

chronic stress;

consumption of foods that contain antibiotics or synthetic hormones (that typically includes nonorganic dairy products, poultry, or meat);

poor diet;

sexual contact with an infected person;

sugar consumption; and

the use of antacids, antibiotics, or birth control pills.[37]

Additionally, health conditions like low thyroid function or diabetes can make a person vulnerable to candida infections.

Do You Have a Candida Infection?

Candida overgrowth can have a damaging effect on our health and our immune system. There are many commonly accepted symptoms and health conditions that actually have a *Candida* overgrowth as a causal factor. The list below is not a complete list, but some of the most common signs and symptoms.

Please keep in mind that this quiz is an assessment tool that is intended for educational purposes only and should not replace a physician's assessment, diagnosis, or testing. Keep in mind that these symptoms/conditions can be linked to other health issues so you should always consult a physician to rule out other possible health issues. You may notice that many of the symptoms of a candida infection overlap with the signs of dysbiosis. That's because candida infections are often the cause of dysbiosis in the gastrointestinal tract.

Give yourself one point for each symptom or condition you have experienced within the last few months.

~ General
- chronic fatigue
- skin conditions (acne, eczema, psoriasis)
- sweet cravings
- weight gain

~ Gastrointestinal system
- alternating diarrhea and constipation
- bloating
- gas
- intestinal cramps
- rectal itching

~ Genitourinary system
- frequent bladder infections
- vaginal yeast infections

~ Hormonal system
- endometriosis
- fibroids
- menopausal symptoms
- menstrual irregularities
- PMS

~ Nervous system
- brain fog
- Depression
- irritability
- trouble concentrating

~ Immune system
- allergies
- arthritis
- chemical sensitivities
- lowered resistance to infections

5

Fermented Foods

The Nearly Forgotten Wisdom of Our Ancestors

In this chapter you'll discover:

- the incredible health benefits of probiotic-rich fermented foods;
- the most popular fermented foods;
- what makes yogurt, kefir, sauerkraut, kimchi, miso, and kombucha such great dietary additions;
- the exciting research that proves the many health benefits of fermented foods;
- forty-five ways to add more fermented foods to your diet; and
- the harmful yogurt ingredient that turns your gut bacteria against you.

Our presence on the planet at this time demonstrates the intelligence and strength of generations of our ancestors that came before us. Their arsenal against plagues and pandemics included making and eating a wide variety of fermented foods, including kimchi, miso, sauerkraut, yogurt, and many other cultured creations.

Plenty of solid research supports fermented foods' place in the diets of our ancestors as well as our modern world's most recent health food stars. The simple act of fermenting everyday foods transforms them into delicious superfoods. Transforming regular food such as vegetables, nuts, and beans into fermented delights such as sauerkraut, yogurt, cheese, and kimchi, their health- and immune-building properties magnify.

Exciting new research shows that fermented foods and the beneficial probiotics they contain can have impressive health effects, some of which include boosting our immune systems, increasing our energy levels, and even preventing and healing many diseases. It's no surprise that fermented foods are the hottest topic in the field of healthy eating right now and seem to be growing in popularity.

Let's explore some of the benefits of the most common forms of fermented foods. If you get to the end of this chapter and find yourself wanting more, check out my book *The Cultured Cook* for recipes to make your own yogurt, sauerkraut, kombucha, and much more.

YOGURT: THE CLASSIC

When it comes to fermented foods, yogurt gets all the glory. Clearly, it is the most popular fermented food in the Western world if the many advertisements, commercials, and articles about the health benefits of yogurt are any indication. And while there is no question that yogurt is one of the most commonly enjoyed fermented foods that offers many health benefits, not all yogurt is created equally. Many commercial yogurts are loaded with additives including sugar, high-fructose corn syrup, dyes, and gums, as well as another harmful ingredient that turns your gut microbes against you. (See the box titled "The Food Additive in Yogurt That Turns Your Gut Bacteria against You" that follows.)

While most research has focused on fermented cow's milk yogurt, the same health benefits are likely from nondairy fermented yogurt made from the milks of coconut, soy (choose organic only as soy is heavily genetically modified), almonds, or cashews, provided they contain live probiotic cultures.

If you're selecting dairy yogurt, choose plain, whole-fat yogurt, ideally made with milk from pasture-raised cows (if buying dairy-based yogurt) and devoid of sugary ingredients or fruit, since it also tends to be heavily sweetened. Check labels for an indication of the live bacteria present in your carton. While its mention on the label doesn't guarantee that the yogurt you've selected includes live cultures thanks to possibly unscrupulous companies, more often than not it will accurately indicate whether it does.

Some of the most healthful bacteria found in yogurt include: *L. bulgaricus, L. casei,* and *Streptococcus thermophilus.* You can purchase ready-made yogurt or you can make your own.

There are many great gut-, immune-, and general health-supporting benefits of eating yogurt or dairy-free yogurt with live cultures on a regular basis.

Yogurt consumption may be helpful for those dealing with respiratory viruses. The *British Journal of Nutrition* found that the probiotic strain *L. casei,* found in most yogurt with live cultures, reduces the duration of respiratory infections and severity of nasal congestion linked with these infections among the elderly.[1]

We know that yogurt supports great gut health, which is backed by extensive research. One study published in the *Journal of the American College of Nutrition* assessed the effects of yogurt consumption of a product containing live *L. casei* cultures on common gastrointestinal infections in shift workers.[2] The researchers found that the yogurt consumption reduced the risk of GI infections. Other research published in the *World Journal of Gastroenterology* showed that yogurt consumption helped to fight *H. pylori* infections.[3]

Yogurt consumption may even boost the immune system's ability to fight cancer. Eating yogurt that contains *L. casei* has been found to have anticancer effects in animal studies, according to a study published in the medical journal *Immunobiology.* The research showed that the probiotic strain blocked tumor development or delayed its growth while improving immune response so the body's immune system could attack the tumor. Additionally, it reduced the number of blood vessels that fed the tumor.[4]

The Food Additive in Yogurt That Turns Your Gut Bacteria against You

Before you eat another spoonful of that yogurt, or even that plant-based yogurt, you'll want to keep reading. And you'll also want to flip the container around and check the ingredient list for a commonly used nanoparticle that may turn your gut bacteria into disease-causing microbes.

Titanium dioxide is found in many common foods especially yogurt and vegan yogurt. It is primarily used in food to deepen a color or to make light-colored foods appear whiter.

Sadly, new research shows that this common food additive turns gut bacteria into weapons of disease. I'll share the research, explain its significance, and share common sources of titanium dioxide that are best avoided altogether.

New research in the medical journal *Frontiers in Nutrition* found that the food additive could cause dysbiosis—detrimental changes in gut microbes and inflammation that may lead to disease.[5] And a growing body of research links harmful changes in gut microbes and gut inflammation to many serious chronic diseases. Good health, or bad health, as the case may be, primarily begins in the gut.

The scientists also found that titanium dioxide could contribute to the formation of biofilms in the gut. Biofilms are sticky substances secreted by harmful bacteria to encourage their growth and to prevent the body's immune system from being able to kill the infectious bacteria. Biofilms are often behind resistant infections that are difficult to treat.

The type of gut alterations resulting from ingesting titanium dioxide, such as mucus layer thickness, increased intestinal permeability (which may be a factor in many autoimmune disorders), and biofilms have been implicated in a wide range of diseases, including colitis and colorectal cancer.

Another recent study published in the medical journal *Environmental Science: Nano,* found that the common food additive altered the healthy functioning of cells in the gut, causing inflammation, increased mucus secretion, and disrupting the intestines' natural ability to protect themselves.[6]

Earlier research in the journal *Scientific Reports* found that the food additive also led to the formation of colon cancer tumors.[7]

While titanium dioxide is used in many varieties of dairy and plant-based yogurt, you'll also find it sneaking into other places in your diet. In a study published in *Environmental Science and Technology,* researchers found the metal nanoparticles in common candies, chewing gums, frostings, puddings, chocolates, coffee creamer, lemonade and other beverages, cookies, marshmallows, and donuts.[8]

It is best to avoid titanium dioxide and the foods containing this harmful metal nanoparticle. The best way to do that is to read ingredient labels on food items and avoid those containing it.

But food is not the only place you'll find this harmful ingredient. You'll also find it hidden in many skincare and personal care products. In addition to the wide range of food products that contain nanoparticles of metal known as titanium dioxide, many consumer products also contain this harmful ingredient, including: cosmetics, toothpastes, sunscreens, creams and lotions, shampoos, deodorants, shaving creams. Even pharmaceutical drugs often contain this suspect ingredient.

Titanium dioxide may also be harmful if it is absorbed through your skin into your bloodstream. While most skincare and beauty products don't list ingredients on their labels, it is best to seek out natural options that clearly indicate that they don't use these types of nanoparticles. There are some excellent natural products, but since the word *natural* isn't adequately regulated, please be advised that many companies may claim that their products are natural even if they contain this toxic ingredient. Ideally, look for personal care and cosmetic products with full disclosure, in the form of ingredient lists, on their packaging.

Regardless of whether you're exposed to titanium dioxide from yogurt, other food items in your diet, or from personal care products, it is best avoided for a healthy gut and immune system.

KEFIR: YOGURT'S HEALTHIER LITTLE SISTER

While yogurt may be the most common fermented food to increase the varieties and populations of probiotics in your intestines, it is certainly not the only, and definitely not the best way, to boost your microbiome. There are many other excellent fermented foods, most of which offer higher amounts and greater diversity of microbes.

Few people have heard about kefir (pronounced ke-FEER), which is a drinkable form of yogurt that offers even greater health benefits. Like yogurt, kefir is a cultured cow's milk product (although there are non-dairy and juice varieties, as well) that has a tart, tangy, sour taste and a slightly bubbly characteristic.

Kefir comes from the Turkish word *keif,* which means "good feeling," probably for the health benefits it offers. This beverage originated in the Caucasus Mountains of Eastern Europe. Thinner in consistency than yogurt, it is made with kefir grains—not actually grains, but a combination of various beneficial bacteria and yeasts. Like yogurt, many commercial kefir products are heavily sweetened and flavored, so be sure to read labels if you're buying premade kefir and choose low-sugar options with the fewest possible ingredients.

Research published in the journal *Biomedicine and Pharmacotherapy* found that kefir and the microorganisms it contains can modulate the immune system to suppress viral infections. It works by activating multiple immune system cells including: B cells, T cells, neutrophils, and cytokines. Although kefir consumption boosts cytokines, the scientists found that kefir's anti-inflammatory activity may also prevent cytokine storms, suggesting that the beverage and its microbes may regulate the immune system to protect against viruses while also protecting against immune system overactivity.[9]

Another study published in the journal *Frontiers in Nutrition* reinforced the findings that kefir consumption helped to balance microbes in the gut and regulated low-grade inflammation. Additionally, the study also found that it reduced gut permeability,[10] or leaky gut, which we discussed earlier as a potential threat to immune system and overall health.

These gut- and immune-balancing effects help to support overall health and may play a role in the many other health benefits attributed to kefir consumption, including heart health, metabolism support, and anticancer effects.

The probiotic *Lactobacillus kefiranofaciens* has been found to produce a substance known as *kefiran*. In a study published in the journal *Biofactors,* researchers found that kefiran from kefir prevented increases in blood pressure, reduced cholesterol levels, and lowered blood sugar levels in animals.[11]

In another study presented in the *International Journal of Obesity,* researchers assessed the effects of kefir consumption on fatty liver disease. Fatty liver disease is a common problem linked with overweight and obesity, insulin resistance, and diabetes. They found that daily kefir consumption improved fatty liver syndrome, and also yielded improvements on specific metabolic issues linked with the disease including increasing metabolic rate, improving energy expenditure, and decreasing triglyceride and cholesterol in the liver.[12]

Probiotics found in kefir also hold promise in the treatment of cancer. One type of probiotic called *Lactobacillus kefiri* was shown to help destroy human leukemia cells even when multiple cancer drugs were unable to induce the cancer cell-killing process. The scientists concluded that the novel kefir bacteria "may act as a potential therapy for the treatment of multidrug-resistant leukemia."[13]

SAUERKRAUT: THE SUPER HEALER

Sauerkraut—fermented cabbage—is not just for hot dogs anymore. In addition to its deliciously tart taste, exciting research showcases the many gut and immune health benefits, among other benefits, of eating sauerkraut (provided it contains live cultures) on a regular basis.

Once again, quality is everything when it comes to beneficial bacteria. Many commercial products use shortcuts, pickling products with white vinegar rather than fermentation, and still more are pasteurized with heat high, which kills any beneficial bacteria that may have been present in the sauerkraut. Make sure to purchase unpasteurized sauerkraut made with traditional fermentation (check farmers markets or the refrigerator sections of natural food stores) or make your own.

Sauerkraut is delicious on its own, atop any kind of sausage, on black bean burgers, or as a side dish to accompany just about any type of meal. While its delicious taste is enough reason to love sauerkraut, its health benefits make it an excellent choice to enjoy on a regular basis.

Regular sauerkraut consumption may be helpful to ward off food poisoning. Research in the journal *Microbiology and Immunology* shows probiotics found in sauerkraut demonstrate antibacterial activity against harmful bacteria, including *Salmonella* and *Shigella*. *Salmonella* can cause food poisoning. *Shigella* are similar bacteria that also cause diarrhea, fever, and stomach cramps.[14]

What if I told you sauerkraut contains beneficial bacteria that are actually miniature antifungal manufacturing facilities? It's true. Some of the probiotics in sauerkraut produce compounds that will kill some species of *Candida* fungi, which are frequently involved in vaginal or intestinal infections. In research published in the *Journal de Mycologie Medicale,* scientists found that the probiotics actually produced antifungal compounds that kill *Candida*.[15]

According to research published in *Current Sports Medicine Reports,* scientists found numerous sports-performance benefits of eating probiotic-rich foods, including improving immune function, as well as reducing allergic conditions and enhancing recovery from fatigue.[16]

In a study published in the journal *Nutrients,* researchers found a link between sauerkraut consumption and a reduction in gastrointestinal symptom severity, as well as immune modulating and enhancing benefits, immune cell activation, and anti-inflammatory effects.[17]

There are still more reasons to love sauerkraut, one of the best superfoods available to boost our health. Sauerkraut consumption has been shown to boost levels of superoxide dismutase and glutathione peroxidase, powerful antioxidants that protect the heart against cellular damage from free radicals.[18] Additionally, scientists found that regularly eating fermented cabbage can help regulate estrogen levels.[19] Excess estrogen levels have been linked with the development of estrogen-dependent breast cancers.

KIMCHI: THE GUT- AND IMMUNE-BOOSTING CONDIMENT

The national dish of Korea, kimchi is a fermented mixture of cabbage, chilies, and garlic, with nearly as many variations as there are Koreans who make it. Used as a condiment in Korea, it can be served alongside or on top of any Asian-inspired dish. Like sauerkraut, it makes an excellent sour, palate-cleansing side alongside nearly any dish.

Scientists have identified a whopping 970 distinct bacterial strains in kimchi.[20] Compare that with the one or two, or occasionally three, strains of probiotics found in most brands of yogurt. Keep in mind that not all kimchi contains 970 different strains of beneficial microbes, but there is definitely a much larger diversity in unpasteurized kimchi that contains live cultures compared to yogurt, which gets all the gut-boosting credit.

One strain in particular, *L. plantarum,* is a research-proven antioxidant. Free radicals are unstable molecules that can damage healthy cells and tissues; antioxidants neutralize free radicals, thereby preventing them from damaging healthy cells. In a study published in the online medical journal *PLOS One,* the probiotic *L. plantarum* demonstrated antioxidant activity stronger than any other probiotic.[21]

Research at Georgia State University found that that same probiotic *L. plantarum* confers protection against the flu by regulating the body's immunity and demonstrating antiviral activity.[22]

Other research on animals found that kimchi consumption resulted in an increase in gut microbial diversity. Other research published in the *Journal of Medicinal Food* found that kimchi consumption even helped to regulate the cytokine process,[23] which may reduce the likelihood of dangerous viral-induced cytokine storms.

In addition to the many immune and gut-health benefits of regularly eating kimchi, research published in the *Journal of Applied Microbiology* found that *L. plantarum* showed potent ability to protect the brain against memory loss in animals. Don't worry, you don't have to remember its name to benefit from its memory-protective effects, but it is good to remember that kimchi is the only food source of this particular probiotic strain, at least that has been identified to date. The scientists concluded that kimchi and this probiotic "may be beneficial for dementia."[24]

Be sure to choose unpasteurized kimchi with a label indicating it "contains live cultures." Look for it in the refrigerator section of health food or grocery stores, not in the middle aisles of grocery stores on unrefrigerated shelves as the latter will have been pasteurized, even if it does not state this on the label. Of course, unsprayed or organic options are best. Pesticides used in the growing of vegetables significantly reduce the beneficial bacterial counts in fermented foods. If you're vegetarian or vegan, you may wish to choose kimchi made without fish sauce, which is a common ingredient in kimchi.

MISO: DELICIOUS IMMUNE REGULATOR

Not just for soup, miso's proven radiation protection means this Japanese staple should warrant further use in our diet. Usually made from fermented soybeans, although you can also find rice and chickpea miso, this mashed ferment is rich in vitamins, minerals, protein, healthy carbs, and, of course, probiotics.

There are many health benefits of enjoying miso on a regular basis. In a large population-based study that took place over fifteen years, researchers found a link between the regular consumption of fermented soybeans and all-cause mortality. They found that a higher intake of fermented soy foods correlated with the lowest risk of mortality. They did not find the same link with unfermented soy foods.[25]

Miso tends to have a high probiotic content, and like other fermented soy products, regular intake has been linked to improved intestinal health.[26] Fermented soy increases the abundance of the probiotics in the Bifidobacteria family, among other probiotics. Research shows that daily intake of fermented soy, such as miso, may contribute to the prevention of inflammation.[27]

Soy contains compounds called flavones, which have been found in animal studies to work on the various cells of the immune system and help to regulate the immune hyperactivity linked with allergic inflammation.[28] Studies have demonstrated that these compounds found in miso may regulate immune responses, suggesting that regular consumption of miso may be helpful for those suffering from allergies.

Another study published in the *International Journal of Molecular Medicine* found that another compound found in soy products, including miso, known as genistein, may help to regulate inflammatory cytokines produced by the immune system and may hold promise in the treatment of allergic inflammation and anaphylactic shock. Of course, that doesn't mean that you should rely on miso as a treatment if you're experiencing anaphylactic shock but should instead seek emergency medical intervention.[29]

As an added bonus, regular consumption of miso has been linked with some protection against radiation injury and the prevention or treatment of lung, liver, breast, and colon cancers.[30]

Keep in mind that many, if not all, of the probiotic bacteria found in miso may be lost when it is heated, such as during the making of miso soup, which is the most common way of eating miso. Miso can be enjoyed in other ways, including being added to salad dressings or blended with raw, soaked cashews to make a delicious dip.

KOMBUCHA: MORE THAN HEALTHY SODA

Kombucha (pronounced kom-BOO-shuh although many people also pronounce it as kom-BOO-chuh, which seems to have become acceptable practice as well) is a beverage believed to have been made in Russia and China for over two thousand years, although the exact origin is unknown. The bacteria and yeasts that form the kombucha culture form a type of "floating mat" on the surface of the tea from which it is typically made. Little research has been done to test the many anecdotal and folkloric claims of its immune-boosting properties, but most of the people I've recommended it to who drink it regularly have reported improved gut health. Some of the reports I've heard, and some of which I've personally experienced as well, include reduced bloating, improved digestion, reduced indigestion, and discomfort. Some people report improved energy, vitality, and immunity, but these are not yet assessed through scientific research, as far as I know.

One study published in the journal *Nutrients* found that kombucha demonstrated significant antioxidant activity against harmful free radicals.[31] Considering that free radicals are linked to aging and disease, this benefit alone makes it worth enjoying this delicious beverage.

Kombucha and its mild carbonation makes a delicious alternative to sugar- and additive-laden soda. While it is made with sugar, minimal sugar is left in the final kombucha beverage, as the sugar becomes food for the probiotics. There are many varieties available on the market, including some that contain excessive levels of sugar, so be sure to read the labels on the variety you select. Also, if you don't like one, there is a huge range of different tastes, so it is worth considering a different option until you find one you like. Ideally, you can also make kombucha at home. It's easy and enjoyable to make your own healthy soda.

Our ancestors knew how to keep their immune systems strong and boost their overall health using fermented food. That's why they incorporated these delicious and nutritious foods into their diet on a regular basis. It's time to follow their lead by adding fermented foods like yogurt, kefir, sauerkraut, kimchi, and kombucha into our diet. You'll discover forty-five ways to do so in the next chapter.

6

The Seven-Step Plan

In chapter 6, you will discover more powerful natural ways to heal the gut, restore microbial balance, and boost your immune system against pathogenic invaders using the best evidence-based gut-healing foods, herbs, oils, nutritional supplements, and more.

You'll discover:

- my Seven-Step Plan for a Great Gut and Super-Powered Immunity and how to incorporate it into your life;
- the most overlooked and affordable way to increase gut microbial diversity—simply feeding gut microbes that are already in your gut or in your diet;
- the most powerful anti-infectious remedies to overcome gut dysbiosis, or microbial imbalances in your gut;
- the best remedies to eliminate yeast infections;
- the best remedies to heal a damaged or leaky gut; and
- herbs like aloe vera, cinnamon, licorice, magnesium, oregano, and how they can help you heal your gut.

If you are dealing with harmful microbial overgrowth or a candida infection, a leaky gut, lowered immunity, or gastrointestinal issues, you will likely benefit from the Seven-Step Plan for a Great

Gut and Super-Powered Immunity. It is a multifaceted approach that addresses many gut-health issues at the same time while also working to rebuild and heal the gut and boosting microbial diversity. You can take a week or even a few weeks to integrate all of the steps of the plan into your daily life if that's what is easiest for you. Regardless of how long it takes you, it is best to stick with the plan for at least four weeks,* but longer if necessary to address long-term gut-health issues, persistent gut infections, or compromised immunity. However, if you're suffering from a serious bowel condition like Crohn's disease or colitis, or bowel cancer, this plan, or components of it, might not be advisable. It is best to check with your doctor before undertaking a new dietary or lifestyle program.

⌇ Overview of the Plan ⌇

Step One: Eliminate Harmful Microbes: Using key herbs, essential oils, and nutrients, as well as a reduced-sugar diet, you'll help address harmful gut microbial imbalances, including candida infections in the gut.

Step Two: Add Fermented Foods to Boost Diversity: Incorporating more probiotics through the addition of at least two different fermented foods to your daily diet increases microbial diversity in your gut, and as we've learned diversity is one of the keys to great health.

Step Three: Boost Probiotics: By adding two capsules of probiotics or one teaspoon of probiotic powder to your daily regime, twice daily, you inoculate your gut with high doses of key beneficial bacteria and yeasts that fight harmful microbes while also helping to heal the gut. By taking them first thing in the morning as well as in the evening on an empty stomach with a glass of water, you'll help ensure they reach the gut to work their magic.

---

*Be mindful that most remedies should not be used for more than three weeks, with a week off afterward.

Step Four: Feed Your Beneficial Microbes: Feeding beneficial microbes helps to boost their ability to proliferate. Adding at least two servings of key prebiotic foods like apples, Jerusalem artichokes, leeks, onions, garlic, chicory root, asparagus, bananas, dandelions, endive, radicchio, burdock, tomatoes, and walnuts, you'll ensure the beneficial microbes have the food they need to proliferate, further helping to eliminate harmful microbes.

Step Five: Water Your Beneficial Microbes: Drinking at least one-half quart or one-half liter of water for every fifty pounds of weight you're carrying, up to three quarts or liters daily, helps to ensure beneficial microbes have the water they need and harmful ones are removed from the body as they are destroyed. Ideally, drinking unchlorinated water or water that has been filtered, even through an inexpensive water pitcher that filters chlorine, prevents the killing of beneficial microbes.

Step Six: Eat a Gut-Supportive Diet: Eating a diet rich in high-fiber fruit, vegetables, nuts, seeds, and legumes further feeds beneficial microbes and helps to eliminate harmful ones as they are destroyed. Ideally, aim for 35 grams total per day.

Step Seven: Heal the Gut Lining: Heal the lining of the intestines to prevent further infections and the release of toxic material into the bloodstream using probiotics and gut-healing herbs.

Now that you have an overview of the plan, let's explore it in greater detail, step by step.

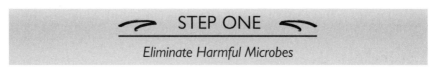

STEP ONE
Eliminate Harmful Microbes

Before we can begin to heal the gut and transform it for super-powered immunity, we need to address any harmful microbial imbalances that may reside in your gut. That includes any possible harmful bacterial or candida fungal infections you may be experiencing. The best way to do so is through the addition of key antimicrobial herbs and nutrients. Let's explore the best antimicrobial remedies for the gut.

There are many great natural remedies that kill *Candida* and other harmful microbes in the intestines. Here are some excellent, all-natural, proven antimicrobials that, when used along with probiotics, a diet that supports the growth of beneficial microbes (outlined in Step Six, which follows), adequate water, and other factors that we'll discuss momentarily, help address an underlying infection that may be having disastrous effects on your health.

Keep in mind that it is important to use whichever remedy or remedies you select on a daily basis until the infection is resolved, usually up to three weeks. It has been my experience that these foods and remedies typically need to be used three times a day every day until the infection is gone. Some of the best natural antimicrobials to help eliminate harmful gut infections, including yeast infections, include coconut oil, dandelion, garlic, olive leaf, and oregano oil. You can learn more about these herbs and others that boost the immune system in my book *Super-Powered Immunity: Natural Remedies for 21st Century Viruses and Superbugs*. Some remedies should not be taken for more than about three weeks, so it is best to immediately switch to another antimicrobial remedy at that time rather than discontinue all antimicrobial remedies.

If you suspect that you may have had gut dysbiosis or *Candida* overgrowth for a long time, you may need to stick with the antimicrobials for a month or two to address any issues. Of course, if you start to experience symptoms again, you'll need to continue with them for a longer period of time.

Coconut Oil

Research at Nigeria's University College Hospital found that coconut oil kills close to 100 percent of yeast cells (even drug-resistant species) on contact thanks to its lauric, caprylic, and capric acid content. These compounds cause the protective outer wall of yeast cells to split apart, making it easier for the immune system to destroy them. The study dose was 3 tablespoons of extra virgin coconut oil daily.[1]

You may be thinking: "That's a lot of coconut oil" or "Isn't coconut oil bad for my health?" Since the American Heart Association (AHA) stated that coconut oil is harmful to health, many people have dropped their favorite cooking oil in favor of canola oil. After all, the AHA recommended the latter as a supposedly healthier option indicating that cooking with coconut oil was just as unhealthy as cooking with butter, beef fat, or bacon fat.[2] It might be tempting to adhere to the AHA advisory, believing that coconuts, and the oil extracted from them, are villains that stalk us from grocery store shelves just waiting to clog our arteries and force us into premature death from heart attack or stroke. But is coconut oil really the enemy of health, or was the AHA advisory just an alarmist perspective on an otherwise healthy oil? What is a person to believe?

Not all saturated fats were created equally. Declaring butter, bacon fat, beef fat, and coconut oil (the latter of which is approximately 82 percent saturated fat) as evil is really an oversimplification of things. On the flip side, the AHA also advised eating more oils from nuts, seeds, and avocado, as well as corn, canola, and soy. The latter three foods, and the oils derived from them, are heavily genetically modified and usually contain the harmful pesticide glyphosate, and as a result are best avoided.

But let's get back to coconut oil. The AHA indicates that consuming coconut oil will increase LDL cholesterol (often called the "bad" cholesterol) and adds that the oil has no qualities that offset its damaging effects. The reality is: coconut oil can raise LDL cholesterol right alongside HDL cholesterol (frequently called the "good" cholesterol). Research shows that consuming coconut oil increases HDL cholesterol and can contribute to reduced abdominal fat—a factor that is a well-documented contributor to heart disease. In other words, consuming coconut oil may actually be beneficial to improve two factors linked to heart disease.[3]

But what about the potential increase in LDL cholesterol? The jury is still out on how harmful it is to heart health. While some experts claim it is the nemesis of heart health, others cite the importance of cholesterol to manufacture essential hormones needed for health. The debate continues, and there is truth to both camps. While cholesterol shouldn't be completely ignored as bloggers across the internet seem to be recommending, neither should it be quite so feared. We need cholesterol to survive (after all, it is the direct precursor of cortisol, which is needed for life, as well as for arterial repair) but we don't need it in excessive quantities either.

Of course, you'll need to make the best decision for you but, provided it makes sense for you considering other health factors, cooking with coconut oil for at least a few weeks may be helpful to address harmful gut microbes. You replace whatever cooking oil you normally use with coconut oil, being sure to cook with it only on low to medium temperatures to avoid smoking. After oils smoke, they are denatured, no longer healthy options, and should therefore not be eaten. And, if you decide that coconut oil isn't right for you, simply select another antimicrobial remedy that follows.

Curcumin (from Turmeric)

Curcumin is an extract of the yellow spice, turmeric, that gives curries their characteristic yellow color and a hint of flavor.

According to a study published in the journal *BioMed Research International,* scientists found that curcumin demonstrated potent antibacterial and antifungal activity against two dozen harmful bacteria it was tested against, making it a good choice in addressing harmful microbial overgrowth in the gut as well as making it a great option to address dysbiosis, particularly when multiple harmful bacteria may be involved in the gut. Among the various bacteria tested, curcumin demonstrated effectiveness against the frequently drug-resistant *Helicobacter pylori* (*H. pylori*), which is often implicated in ulcers and gastrointestinal health issues. The study also showed that curcumin demonstrated potent antifungal activity including against *Candida albicans,* making it a good option if you have, or suspect that you might have, a *Candida* overgrowth. Curcumin was even effective against a range of *Candida* strains that are frequently resistant to the drug fluconazole.[4]

Garlic

A natural antibiotic, antifungal, and antiviral agent, garlic is rich in the immune-boosting and antimicrobial sulfur compound known as allicin, making it a great addition to your diet.

Research published in the journal *Microbes and Infection* found garlic demonstrated high antibacterial activity against a range of harmful bacteria, including drug-resistant strains of *E. coli* that can inhabit the gut and elsewhere in the body, it also exerted potent antifungal activity against *Candida albicans.*[5]

Garlic is most antibacterial and antifungal when eaten raw, but cooked garlic is still a worthy dietary addition, both for flavor and its antimicrobial benefits. Ideally, eat one raw clove of garlic daily. Garlic is also readily available in capsule form, usually as standardized allicin extracts. For these preparations, a therapeutic dose would be 600–900 milligrams of garlic, yielding 6 milligrams of allicin daily, but it is best to follow the package directions for the product you select, since potency and dosage size can vary between products.

While garlic plays an important role in restoring microbial balance to the gut, excessive garlic consumption can irritate the intestinal tract, causing nausea, diarrhea, or vomiting, as well as burning of the mouth. Add raw garlic to previously cooked foods just prior to eating or throw it in a homemade salad dressing and enjoy atop leafy greens, steamed vegetables, or a baked sweet potato. Toss some fresh, chopped garlic into your favorite soup, stew, chili, stir-fry, or meat or veggie dish. And you can also enjoy raw garlic in hummus by mixing it with chickpeas, tahini (sesame puree), lemon juice, olive oil, and a dash of salt. It is best to leave garlic powder behind since most of its health benefits are long gone; however, if fresh garlic is unavailable, it is better than no garlic at all.

It is best avoided or eaten in only small quantities among those taking anticoagulant drugs, such as blood thinners. Consult your physician if you are taking these drugs before consuming high amounts of garlic or garlic capsules.[6]

German Chamomile (*Matricaria chamomilla* or *Matricaria recutita*)

While German chamomile is not typically among my top selections for antimicrobial remedies, the herbal remedy has demonstrated specific effectiveness with candida infections, and therefore warrants a brief mention and consideration if you're dealing with a candida infection. While the remedy may be helpful in such cases, it should not be used on its own to address microbial overgrowth or candida infections. It is best to pair it with at least one or two other remedies for best results.

Researchers assessed the antimicrobial activity of an extract of German chamomile against the fungus *Candida albicans*. According to the *Indian Journal of Dentistry*, a high-potency extract of chamomile effectively killed the fungal infection.[7] While the study examined the oral use of the remedy against the infection, it is likely that the benefits would be found in the gut as well when used to address candida infections.

While chamomile's flowers may seem an unlikely source for such impressive antimicrobial effects, the delicate flowers should not be underestimated. They can be used fresh or dried and kept in a jar and brewed into a tea. Pre-packaged chamomile tea is also readily available in most health food and grocery stores. Chamomile is also available in alcohol-based tinctures or glycerin-based glycerites—which are a better choice for those who cannot use alcohol, as well as for children. Since chamomile is in the same family as ragweed, it is best avoided if you are allergic to ragweed. Also, the drug warfarin (Coumadin) has been found to interact with chamomile. Other blood thinners may also interact with chamomile, so it is best not to use chamomile if you are taking these drugs. Consult your physician prior to use if you are taking these or other drugs.

A chamomile infusion of one to two teaspoons of herb per cup of boiled water can be brewed for ten minutes and drunk for internal use. Alternatively, brew the infusion in the same manner, allow to cool, and use as a mouthwash for dental or oral health issues. It can be covered and stored in the fridge for up to three days.

Olive Leaf

In ancient Egypt, olive leaves were deemed a symbol of heavenly power[8] and were first used medicinally. Since then, olive leaf has become valued worldwide for its many therapeutic uses, particularly for infectious conditions.

The leaves of olive trees contain powerful antioxidants and are anti-inflammatory, but perhaps they hold their greatest value in their anti-infectious ability. Olive leaves contain a compound known as oleuropein that is abundant in both the leaves as well as the olives and is believed to be responsible their many healing properties. Doctors at the Department of Biomedical Science at CHA University in Korea found that olive leaf extract was potent against various microbes. Additionally, their research showed olive leaf exhibited free radical scavenging abilities.[9] Other research also supports olive leaf's broad antimicrobial activity against bacteria, viruses, and fungi, including candida infections.[10]

Available in many forms from health food stores, including extracts, dried leaf or teabags, or capsules, you can select the olive leaf extract that best suits your needs and desired method of delivery. If you have oral candida infection, select either a toothpaste, mouthwash, or a liquid extract that is suitable for swishing in your mouth for a few minutes. For gut or systemic infections, the easiest way to obtain olive leaf is through an extract, either a tincture or another liquid product on the market. Use 1 to 2 milliliters of a tincture, three times daily. Olive leaf is also available in capsules ranging between 500 to 1,000 milligrams daily. Ideally divide the dose two to three times daily, up to 1,000 milligrams daily, taken with food. Olive leaf tea, while not typically as potent as other forms, is also available in most health food stores, and is still worth using. Regardless which type of product you select, follow the package directions for use.

Olive leaf tends to be safe for most uses; however, there are some safety considerations. Those with low blood pressure may need to exercise caution as it can reduce blood pressure and cause dizziness. It may irritate the stomach if the dose is too high; dilute with water or reduce the dosage in that case. It can cause diarrhea, acid reflux, headaches, heartburn, or stomach pain in some people. Avoid use if you're pregnant or breastfeeding, except under the guidance of a physician. Avoid use with blood pressure medications. If you are taking medications for diabetes, it is advisable to check with your physician, and if he or she agrees, to start with small amounts of olive leaf extract. Olive leaf extract may boost the effects of blood-thinning drugs like warfarin, so you'll want to check with your physician prior to using and be monitored throughout use, if he or she agrees. Olive leaf may also interact with some chemotherapy drugs, so it is best to check with your physician prior to use.[11]

Oregano (*Origanum vulgare*)

The King of natural antibiotics, study after study proves the effectiveness of oregano oil. Of course, like anything, product strength can vary drastically. Some products are actually marjoram and not oregano at all, and thanks to them both being part of the scientific family Origanum, it's easy to confuse the two, but manufacturers should know the difference and select *Origanum vulgare,* since it is true oregano and is therapeutic for the intended antibacterial and antiviral effects. Ideally, choose a reputable brand backed by independent research.

Dozens of scientific sources show that oregano has demonstrated significant antioxidant activity, making it effective in preventing or alleviating many health conditions caused or aggravated by the presence of free radicals in the body.

Research reported in the journal *Microbial Ecology in Health and Disease* showcased oregano's antibacterial activity and effectiveness against two types of bacteria, in particular *Klebsiella oxytoca* and *Klebsiella pneumonia*.[12] These bacteria can infect the skin, wounds, throat, gastrointestinal tract, urinary tract, and particularly the lungs.[13]

In addition to the effectiveness against the bacteria mentioned above, research published in the journal *Frontiers in Microbiology* showcased the effectiveness of oregano against antibiotic-resistant strep infections, particularly strep throat. This study used oregano essential oil, which is a particularly potent extract of the oil components of the plant.[14]

Oregano has also been found effective against candida infections. New research in the medical journal *MicrobiologyOpen* found that oregano worked against six different strains of *Candida* fungus.[15]

Oregano is available in fresh or dried herb, essential oil, capsule, or tincture formats. Add the fresh or dried herb to your soups, salads, stews, curries, or other savory foods. While adding it to foods is certainly beneficial, you may need higher doses than that which is available in food. In the case of infectious conditions, use oregano essential oil, which is often simply called oregano oil, making sure that the one you select is suitable for internal use. Additionally, you may also find oregano oil capsules or gel capsules easier to take. And, of course, oregano extract in a tincture (alcohol extract) form is also beneficial. Follow package directions for the essential oil, capsule, or tinctures you select.

Thyme (*Thymus vulgaris*)

Few people think of thyme when they seek antimicrobial remedies to deal with gut overgrowth, which is a shame because it is one of the best options.

In a study published in the *Journal of Microbiology and Biotechnology* assessing the effectiveness of thyme and oregano, as well as basil, essential oils against harmful microbes, researchers found that all three were effective against a wide variety of bacterial stains. In their assessment of the essential oils' effects on *E. coli,* the researchers found that both thyme and oregano were the most effective.[16] Research published in the scientific journal, *Molecules,* found that thyme, as well as oregano, demonstrated the greatest effectiveness against the harmful gut bacteria *E. coli* and as well as the fungi *Candida albicans* and *Candida famata.*[17]

What's more, a study published in the *Brazilian Journal of Microbiology* found that not only was thyme effective at inhibiting fungal growth, but it also increased the ability of the drug fluconazole to kill the disease-causing fungi.[18] That's good news for *Candida* sufferers, since this is a drug that is often prescribed to treat the fungal overgrowth. Regardless of whether you opt for drugs or if you prefer a natural approach, you'll be happy to know that a study published in the journal *BMC Complementary and Alternative Medicine* found that thyme was even effective against drug-resistant strains of *Candida.*[19]

The late herbal medicine pioneer and author of *The Green Pharmacy,* James A. Duke, Ph.D., recommended using one teaspoon of dried thyme per cup of boiled water and steeping the herb for about ten to fifteen minutes to make thyme tea. Drink three cups daily for maximum effectiveness.[20] Of course, you can also add thyme to meat, poultry, vegetable, and legume dishes with a side of antimicrobial benefits.

Two to three drops of pure therapeutic grade thyme essential oil can be added to empty capsules and taken three times daily to help prevent or address infections. Be sure that the product you select is suitable for internal use and preferably one with third-party laboratory verification attesting to its purity. Use thyme or thyme essential oil with caution during pregnancy. Dilute heavily for topical use or for oral use if you have gastrointestinal issues. Thyme is also available in a tincture form. Use approximately 2 to 4 milliliters three times daily. Follow directions for the product you select.

I'm unaware of any drug interactions with thyme, other than its ability to increase the effectiveness of fluconazole, but if you're taking any medications or have any health issues, it's best to consult with your physician prior to use.

North American Ginseng (*Panax quinquefolius L.*)

While ginseng is most known for its vitality-boosting and immune-enhancing effects, it is also a good choice for eliminating harmful microbes in the gut. But no one would argue with the desirable side effects of added vitality and immunity when dealing with candida infections, which is supported by research. In an animal study published in the *Journal of Ethnopharmacology* researchers found that ingestion of Panax ginseng, as it is often called, significantly reduced *Candida albicans* infection.[21] So you may wish to include ginseng in the herbs you select if you're dealing with a candida infection or if you feel a general malaise and low vitality that may be affecting your immune system and overall health.

ANTIMICROBIAL HERBAL REMEDIES

Herbal Remedy	Method of Use
Garlic	Capsule, Fresh Herb (baking, cooking), Tincture
Ginseng (Panax/North American)	Dried Herb, Tea, Extract, Tincture
Olive Leaf	Dried Herb, Tea, Extract, Tincture
Oregano	Capsule, Dried Herb (baking, cooking), Tea, Tincture, Essential Oil
Thyme	Dried Herb, Tea, Essential Oil

Extracts of the above herbs are widely available in health food stores. A typical tincture dose for the above herbal medicines is 30 drops three times daily taken under the tongue. Because drug–herb interactions and medical contraindications are common, it is best to follow package instructions for the product you select and consult your physician regarding any possible conditions you may have and drugs you may be taking. Follow the guidelines for internal use of essential oils, as most oils are not suitable for this purpose.

STEP TWO

Add Fermented Foods to Boost Diversity

Microbial diversity is one of the keys to great health, as you may have guessed from the information and studies shared throughout *Super-Powered Immunity Starts in the Gut*. One of the best ways to boost diversity is to add more fermented foods to your diet. Ideally, strive to eat at least two different varieties every day.

And, as you discovered, even the best yogurt is unlikely to provide a wide range of different microbes, but it is still a good way to obtain some key strains in beneficial quantities. In other words, it's a great idea to eat yogurt, but it's also wise to go beyond yogurt.

In addition to yogurt, enjoy kefir, sauerkraut, kimchi, miso, kombucha, and many other fermented foods as part of your daily diet and you'll reap the rewards of microbial diversity, some of which include better digestion and gut health, stronger immunity, and even a healthier body weight.

If you're like many people, you may not know how to get more fermented foods into your diet, outside of yogurt with fruit or sauerkraut on your favorite hot dog. Here are forty-five of my favorite ways to get more fermented foods into your diet. Of course, don't feel constrained by the list. Feel free to experiment with fermented foods. You might just find some novel ways of incorporating them into your diet. Here are some ideas to get you started:

Using Yogurt or Kefir

1. Atop Pancakes or Waffles—Add a dollop of yogurt along with some fresh or frozen (thawed, of course) fruit instead of or in addition to maple syrup.

2. Snack on a delightful traditional Greek dish—yogurt served with a drizzle of honey and walnuts.

3. As the Basis of Dips—Swap out the typical sour cream used in many dips with yogurt and enjoy the probiotic health benefits of doing so. Add herbs like chopped spring onions, basil, thyme, garlic, or others for a delicious spinach dip.

4. Smoothies—Blend fresh or frozen berries with some yogurt or kefir for a probiotic-powered smoothie.

5. Frozen Yogurt—After making a fruit smoothie, pour it into popsicle molds for a frozen yogurt treat.

6. Breakfast Cereal—Reduce the amount of milk or plant-based milk you add to your cereal and stir in a dollop or two of yogurt or kefir to your favorite breakfast cereal or oatmeal.

7. Risotto—After cooking risotto and removing it from the heat, add a dollop or two of yogurt for a taste sensation that's ultra creamy.

8. Yogurt Salad Dressing—Blend some yogurt with lemon juice or vinegar and some herbs and sea salt for a creamy salad dressing.

9. Yogurt Cheese—Line a sieve with cheesecloth, set it atop a bowl or large Pyrex pitcher, pour in some yogurt, and let it sit for at least a few hours to make a soft yogurt cheese. Add fresh herbs for a delicious soft cheese that freshens up any dish or is delicious on its own.

10. Save Yogurt to Make Perpetual Yogurt—Save a few tablespoons of yogurt or the whey from yogurt-making as the starter culture to make even more. That way, you reduce your cost of having perpetually available yogurt.

Using Sauerkraut, Pickled Vegetables, or Kimchi

11. Grilled Cheese—Add well-drained sauerkraut to a grilled cheese (vegan or dairy cheese, whichever you prefer) for a delicious and sour twist.

12. Hummus—Add a can of chickpeas, a splash of olive oil, tahini (pureed sesame seeds), and sauerkraut juice for a quick and probiotic-rich hummus. The sauerkraut juice adds flavor and probi-

otics and replaces some of the salt in this recipe, so be sure to check before adding extra salt.

13. Over Brown Rice or Quinoa for a Quick Meal—When I don't feel up to making dinner, I throw some rice or quinoa into my rice cooker, serve, and top with fermented vegetables for a delicious and nutritious meal in a hurry. By keeping my fridge stocked with various fermented vegetables, I can serve up a gourmet rice bowl with minimal effort.

14. Spinach Dip—Add sauerkraut juice, garlic, and a pinch of sea salt (if necessary, because sauerkraut juice is naturally salty) to yogurt, then stir in a handful or two of steamed or sauteed spinach after it cools for a delicious dip.

15. Tacos—Add naturally fermented onions or mixed fermented vegetables to your tacos for a flavor boost.

16. Salad Dressing—Blend sauerkraut or kimchi with 2 parts oil and 1 part vinegar for a quick and easy salad dressing.

17. Over Salad—Fermented pickles or well-drained sauerkraut (especially the dill-flavored varieties) make a delicious topping for Caesar salads, but they work on other types of salads as well.

18. Over Noodles—Add a couple of spoonfuls of kimchi to vermicelli noodles after draining them for a delicious meal in minutes.

19. Salad Rolls—Soak rice paper wraps in hot water, then pat dry. Add pickled veggies, along with vermicelli noodles, and fresh mint, and wrap for a delicious snack or dinner. Serve with peanut sauce or sweet chili sauce for dipping.

20. Sandwiches—Add fermented onions, pickled turnip, sauerkraut, or kimchi to your favorite sandwich to give it a flavor and nutritional boost.

21 and 22. On Burgers and Hot Dogs—This one is fairly self-explanatory.

23. Lettuce Cups—Add bean sprouts, fermented vegetables, and freshly grated vegetables to a large leaf of lettuce, along with a splash of sweet chili sauce, and wrap it up for a simple snack or meal.

24. Condiments—Add pickled vegetables or kimchi as a condiment to almost any meal.

25. Salsa and Chips—Add the contents of one probiotic capsule to chopped tomatoes, onion, garlic, lemon juice (or a splash of sauerkraut juice), and minced chilies. Cover and let sit for at least a few hours or overnight at room temperature. Serve your fermented salsa with corn chips or other chip for a probiotic-rich snack or party favorite.

26. Guacamole—Add some coarsely chopped fermented vegetables like pickles to mashed avocado for a simple and uniquely delicious guacamole in minutes.

ᦔ Using Miso ᦕ

27. Soup—There's the old standby, miso soup. Ideally, wait until the hot water cools slightly then whisk the miso into it for a soup replete with probiotics left intact.

28. Sandwich Filling—Add a tablespoon or two to chickpeas, as well as some spring onion and a dash of salt, then mash for a delicious sandwich filling.

29. Grain Goodness—Add a couple of tablespoons of miso to the cook water for brown rice, quinoa, or other grain. Alternatively, cook the grains and stir in the miso while they are still warm.

30. Buttery Spread—Over low heat, melt a cup of coconut oil. Once melted, remove from the heat and stir in a couple of tablespoons of miso. Allow to cool, stirring occasionally to ensure even distribution of the miso bits. Use in place of butter when you want a rich, slightly salty, slightly sweet taste.

31. Great Glaze—In a small bowl mix together 2 tablespoons of pure maple syrup, 2 tablespoons of miso (I prefer dark varieties for this recipe), a small fresh chili of your choice (minced), and a tablespoon of olive oil. This Maple Miso Glaze works beautifully on slices of tofu (choose organic only) or over roasted vegetables. For the tofu, cut into half-inch-thick slices and coat with the glaze, then bake at 350 degrees Fahrenheit for about 20 to 25 minutes.

32. Savory Crème Fraîche—Soak raw, unsalted cashews in water overnight. Blend with some miso and just enough of the soak water to produce a thick and creamy cream. Pour over your favorite grains or cooked vegetables.

33. Miso Vinaigrette—In a medium-sized jar add: ⅔ cups olive oil, ⅓ cup rice vinegar, 2 tablespoons miso, and 1 teaspoon agave or maple syrup. Shake all ingredients together in a jar or blend with a hand blender. Toss with greens and serve.

34. Salad Dressing Booster—Instead of using mustard to thicken your homemade salad dressing, use miso. It thickens and emulsifies salad dressings.

35. Vegan Sour Cream Sensation—Add some miso and lemon juice to raw, unsalted cashews soaked in water overnight. Blend together until smooth, adding only enough water to reach a sour cream consistency. Pour over baked potatoes, add to your favorite taco, or use as you would traditional varieties of sour cream.

36. Green Greatness—Sauté your favorite leafy greens in miso, garlic, olive oil, and rice wine vinegar for great greens.

37. Veggie Burger Boost—Spread a thin layer of miso in place of mayo on your next veggie burger for a delicious, salty, rich flavor boost.

38. Mayo or Aioli—Puree some miso with a small amount of water and stir into your favorite aioli or mayo. Spread on sandwiches, subs, or add to wraps.

39. Miso Mustard—Puree some miso with a small amount of water and stir into your favorite hot mustard for a taste treat. Use as you would regular mustard.

40. Stewed Up—Add a tablespoon or two to your favorite stew for a rich flavor boost.

Using Other Fermented Foods

41. Pro-Powered Juice—Empty the contents of a probiotic capsule into your favorite fruit or vegetable juice, cover and leave at room temperature overnight or for a day. Not only will you get the probiotics

found in the capsule, but the beneficial microbes will proliferate and actually reduce the amount of natural sugars present in the juice.

42. Choose Kombucha over Soda—Skip the sugar-laden soft drink and instead enjoy a naturally sparkling kombucha (a probiotic-rich beverage).

43. Cultured Cream—Soak raw, unsalted nuts like cashews, pine nuts, or macadamias in enough water to cover and add the contents of one probiotic capsule. Let sit for 8 hours or overnight. Blend. Use in place of cream on hot chocolate or over fruit bowls. Use only as much of the soak water as needed for a thick vegan sour cream.

44. Vegan Cheese—Follow the instructions under 23 but use only enough water to cover the nuts and allow them to ferment with the probiotic powder for at least 24 hours or longer for a sharper cheese flavor. Blend until smooth and creamy for a quick and probiotic-rich soft cheese.

45. Vegan Cheesecake or Pudding—Follow the instructions for vegan cheese but add some fruit and sweetener (if you wish), along with a couple tablespoons of a thickening agent like ground chia or flax seeds. For a cheesecake, crumble some graham crackers or cookies with a small amount of coconut oil and press into a small cheesecake mold. Pour the fruit-cashew mixture over the crust. Refrigerate until firm, et voila! Enjoy a simple, raw, probiotic-rich pudding or cheesecake.

↶ STEP THREE ↷

Boost Probiotics

Adding a high-quality probiotic supplement to your daily regime can significantly improve your gut and immune health. Here are some tips to help you select a high-quality probiotic supplement.

Factors to Consider when Purchasing Probiotic Supplements

◊ Company Reputation

While there are many companies manufacturing probiotic supplements, some do so simply to capitalize on the growing trend toward taking probiotic supplements. While there may be nothing wrong with a start-up probiotics manufacturing company, ideally select one that offers third-party proof that their product claims are pure and contain the items listed on the product label.

◊ Science-Supported Strains

There are many strains of probiotics but few of them have been adequately researched to warrant supplementation with them. Most people tend to think that more ingredients are superior to fewer ingredients, but a long list of bacterial strains is not necessarily better than a short list of well-researched and proven-effective strains when it comes to health outcomes. Keep in mind that bacteria compete with each other for nutrition and resources, so dominant strains may simply beat out the strains that are less resilient, rendering them useless. So if you're paying more for a product with more probiotic strains than others, you might be throwing your money away. Or you could be paying for strain combinations that are untested through research to accomplish what you want them to, including boosting gut health, fighting infections, and boosting immunity. While the "throw everything into the pool" approach may seem like a good idea, it is rarely effective when it comes to probiotics.

◊ Stability

As I just mentioned, some strains cannot keep pace with more dominant strains, due to their lack of stability. Therefore, inclusion of unstable strains in a supplement is not advisable. Additionally, by the time the product has been manufactured, transported, and sits on store shelves for a period of time before it gets to you, it may no longer contain some of the probiotics reported. There's no easy way for consumers to determine the stability of microbes present in the products they purchase until they've taken them home and attempted to make yogurt from them.

Probiotics are measured in colony forming units, or CFU, which represents the reported number of live bacteria. Product labels usually indicate 1 to 25 billion CFUs of specific probiotic strains. Some companies assert that their product contains 5 billion organisms "at the time of manufacture," which is actually useless information and frankly misleading to consumers.

Probiotics can and do die over time, when exposed to heat or when they are not refrigerated, as well as when they are impacted by other factors. Other companies report the number of organisms at the end of the shelf life of the product, which is actually a much more useful number. Opt for products that report the number of organisms at the end of the shelf life. Companies that report the number of CFUs at the end of the shelf life usually factor in a 50 percent loss of probiotic cultures by the expiration date of the product. In other words, a product that claims to have 10 billion CFUs by the expiration date may actually have many more than that throughout its shelf life. However, as with any type of consumer product there will always be some products that simply do not contain what they claim to contain. Sites like ConsumerLab.com periodically review probiotic supplements, should you wish to find specific brands or products that fare well when tested.

◊ Mixture of Cultures

You'll want a combination of both Lactobacilli and Bifidobacteria since Lactobacilli are more likely to inoculate the small intestines while Bifidobacteria are more likely to inoculate the large intestines, and you'll want both for a healthy gut.

◊ Potency

Most products contain anywhere from one to fifty billion active cultures, although the latter rarely occurs in reality, despite what the label might state, especially when you consider the die-off that occurs from manufacturing until it reaches your body. Most people benefit from one billion CFUs of the specific strains for maintaining general health but in some cases, people may need higher doses.

Should Everyone Supplement with Probiotics?

Probiotics may be beneficial for most people, but they may not be right for everyone at every time in life. And, some probiotic strains are not suitable for certain periods of life, such as infancy or early childhood for example. Additionally, some probiotics can interact with certain medications, and there can be circumstances during which time probiotics may be best avoided.

◊ Contraindications with Some Medications

Some doctors tell their patients that taking probiotics along with antibiotic treatment can reduce the effectiveness of the antibiotics. I haven't seen the research to support that claim and believe that the concern may actually more theoretical in nature than proven fact. On the flip side, I have seen research that demonstrates that probiotics may boost the effectiveness of certain antibiotics. Having said this, if your doctor or pharmacist suggest you avoid probiotics while taking antibiotics, you should follow these instructions.

You may need to avoid probiotic supplements before surgery to prevent any possible blood-thinning effects, as well as after undergoing transplant surgery since you may need to take medications that suppress your immune system. Some of the medications that decrease the immune system include: azathioprine (Imuran), basiliximab (Simulect), cyclosporine (Neoral, Sandimmune), daclizumab (Zenapax), muromonab-CD3 (OKT3, Orthoclone OKT3), mycophenolate (CellCept), tacrolimus (FK506, Prograf), sirolimus (Rapamune), prednisone (Deltasone, Orasone), corticosteroids (glucocorticoids), and others. Check with your doctor or pharmacist if you're not sure, keeping in mind that your doctor may have intended the immune-lowering effects for a purpose.

◊ Other Considerations before Taking Probiotic Supplements

Infants should only use a reputable probiotic formulated for infants. While Lactobacilli are likely safe for most people including babies and children, not all products may be. Use of probiotics during pregnancy and breastfeeding is probably safe, but many strains of probiotics have not been studied for this application so their safety may be unknown, so keep that in mind. The probiotic *Bifidobacterium infantis* is often recommended for infants, as the name would suggest, but you should still check the product and with your physician before using probiotics with infants and children.

Additionally, if a person has a weak immune system, he or she should consult with a physician prior to using probiotics.

◊ Allergies

If you suffer from severe allergies known as anaphylaxis or anaphylaxis reactions, then you'll want to ensure that the product does not contain any of the substances to which you are allergic or that the probiotics have not been grown on something to which you are allergic. If you have a gluten, milk, soy, wheat, corn, or other allergy or sensitivity, be sure to check the label to ensure that it doesn't contain traces of these food products. Keep in mind, however, that there can still be minute trace amounts of dairy products, particularly in Lactobacilli strains, as they are usually extracted from dairy products. If you have a dairy allergy, check the package and choose products that are guaranteed to be free of dairy products.

◊ Storage Methods

How are the supplements stored? Are they in a refrigerator when you buy them or are they sitting on store shelves at room temperature? While it is true that some probiotic strains do not need refrigeration, most do. Cooler temperatures tend to keep probiotics viable for longer periods of time. Ideally, choose products that are stored in the refrigerator, then store them in your fridge when you get them home. Try not to leave them in a hot vehicle or in your purse out in the sunshine for long periods of time. They might be fine for an hour or two but will have lost much of their potency if you leave them there for a weekend during the hot summer months.

◊ Probiotic Supplements Should Never Be One Size Fits All

Certain health issues, including the type of infections you may be dealing with, the status of your gut health or lack thereof, whether or not you've used antibiotics or are still using them, as well as other factors, all play a role in the type of probiotic you may wish to use. For example, *Bifidobacterium* and *Saccharomyces* strains of probiotics seem to have beneficial effects on the harmful bacteria known as *H. pylori*.

The most common probiotic strains you'll find in supplements include: *L. acidophilus, L brevis, L. bulgaricus, L. casei, L. delbrueckii, L. gasseri, L. johnsonii, L. paracasei, L. plantarum, L. reuteri, L. rhamnosus, L. salivarius, B. bifidum, B. breve, B. infantis, B. lactis,* and *B. longum*. As mentioned earlier, that doesn't mean you need all of them for gut or immune health.

I've created a chart that follows to help you to address gut and immune health issues, as well as overcome common infections using probiotics; however, probiotics are not cure-alls, so you should follow the advice of your physician.

And keep in mind that if a store salesperson tells you that he or she has a probiotic product that works on every health problem, I'd seriously question the validity of that statement.

How to Take Probiotic Supplements for the Best Results

It takes time for probiotic supplements to work. Yes, you may feel improvement in your digestive symptoms, nausea, bloating, or diarrhea within thirty minutes of taking them, but you should not expect to see immediate results for healing chronic gut problems. Probiotics go to work on the potential source of your health issues rather than just mask symptoms. That takes time to address and correct what is often many years of neglect or dietary abuse to our digestive system.

Ideally, take probiotic supplements on an empty stomach (although adding them to smoothies and other liquids is fine as these types of foods tend to digest quickly and don't slow the probiotics from getting to the intestines where they ultimately need to be). If you are taking antibiotics or even natural products with antibiotic effects such as oregano oil, olive leaf, and similar supplements mentioned earlier in this chapter, you may wish to take them at different times of day. For most people, the ideal time to take probiotic supplements is either before bed or first thing in the morning. If you take them in the morning, try to leave at least 20 to 30 minutes before eating so they make their way quickly through the digestive tract to reach the intestines where they are desired. Most people benefit from two capsules or a half teaspoon in the morning on an empty stomach. If you're taking probiotic powder you can measure a half teaspoon into water and drink it. Or add it to your smoothie.

If you are suffering from an infectious disease or candida infection, I typically find double dosing (two capsules, twice a day) tends to be effective. If you have a sensitive or irritable gut, or a gut condition, start with the minimum dose recommended on the product label. Of course, if you have a serious infection you should immediately consult a health professional.

Which Probiotic Strains Are Best for You?

The following chart serves as a basic guideline to help you select beneficial probiotic strains for your specific health needs. These are unlikely to be the only effective strains so you may wish to include them in your daily regime as part of a broad-spectrum probiotic. It is unlikely that you will find these individual strains in capsules on their own, but as part of a broader spectrum supplement. This chart is in no way complete as more research on probiotics arrives almost daily. The chart is a starting point to help you select the probiotics that may be beneficial for you.

Condition/Infection	Probiotic Strains Found in Research to Be Effective
Digestion	L. acidophilus and L. plantarum
Antibiotic Use or Diarrhea resulting from Antibiotic use	B. lactis, L. reuteri, L. casei, L. bulgaricus, S. thermophiles, L. acidophilus, L. paracasei, S. thermophiles, S. boulardii
Irritable Bowel Syndrome (IBS) or Gut Inflammation	L. plantarum, L. rhamnosus, B. longum, L. salivarius, Streptococcus thermophiles
Colitis	Streptococcus thermophilus (but check with your doctor first)
H. pylori infection	L. casei, L. reuteri
E. coli infection	L. casei, L. rhamnosus, Saccharomyces boulardii
C. difficile infection	L. gasseri, L. paracasei, L. plantarum, L. rhamnosus, B. bifidum, Saccharomyces boulardii
Listeria infection	L. gasseri
Enterococcus infections (often impact heart, urinary tract, wounds)	L. gasseri
S. aureus infection	L. paracasei
Candida infection	Saccharomyces boulardii

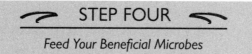

STEP FOUR

Feed Your Beneficial Microbes

In addition to eating a gut-supportive diet, which you will learn about in Step Seven, it is also important to provide beneficial microbes with the foods they love. As a token of gratitude for treating them well, these good bacteria and yeasts will repay you in kind. They will proliferate to magnify their many healing benefits, which include a healthier gut, fewer digestive issues, stronger immunity, and a more balanced immune system, as well as many other potential health benefits, which may include: a healthier respiratory system, a stronger cardiovascular system, fewer allergies, a more balanced body weight, and much more. So, what are the best foods to feed microbes? This is not something most people know about or have even been exposed to.

Prebiotics: Food for the Microbial Troops

Perhaps you never thought about the fact that microbes need food. But it probably comes as no surprise that, like all living things, probiotics need food to survive. You may have even heard of *prebiotics*. Note that is not the same as *probiotics*, which we've already discussed. *Prebiotics* are the group of foods that feed beneficial microbes, thereby enabling them to multiply and populate our gastrointestinal tract. Prebiotics are sugars, starches, and fiber that are found in plant-based foods. Fructooligosaccharides (FOS) and inulin are the two most commonly known types of prebiotics.

Eating more probiotic-rich foods and popping supplements aren't the only ways to increase the populations of beneficial microbes in your intestines. One of the best ways to do so is to add more foods to your diet that beneficial microbes thrive on. Doing so helps to increase their numbers, which in turn offers peripheral benefits to your health and immunity.

Confused? Probiotics vs. Prebiotics: What You Need to Know

Are you confused about probiotics and *prebiotics*? This is a dilemma facing many people, and outrageous marketing claims by many companies seeking to benefit from their popularity aren't helping matters. So, what's the difference?

Just to recap: Probiotics are the microorganisms that promote health. They are primarily bacteria that offer health benefits when eaten or when incorporated into our diet through supplementation. As you learned, there are many different strains of bacteria and some yeasts that offer an array of health benefits, ranging from boosting your gut, strengthening immunity as well as reducing inflammation, boosting brain health, and even helping to fight cancer. These bacteria are primarily from the Lactobacilli and Bifidobacteria families.

*Pre*biotics are the food that probiotics feed on to enable them to populate the intestines. Many food products and supplements come with claims that they contain prebiotics that are necessary for probiotics to work, but that isn't the whole story. While they can be helpful additions to foods, in most cases, adding prebiotics to packaged foods or supplements isn't necessary and is really more of a marketing gimmick. Here's why: *Pre*biotics are found in all plant-based foods in varying amounts. Beneficial bacteria feed on these substances in our gut and proliferate, improving gut health and overall health. If you eat fruit or fiber- and carbohydrate-rich whole grains and beans, your body likely has all the prebiotics it needs to encourage the growth of beneficial microbes in your gut. But you'll still want to make a concerted effort to eat more fermented foods or take probiotic supplements to get adequate probiotics to boost the diversity and populations of beneficial microbes in your gut.

Some of the best sources of prebiotics include: apples, Jerusalem artichokes, leeks, onions, garlic, chicory root, asparagus, bananas, dandelions, endive, radicchio, and burdock. While tomatoes and walnuts are not typically found on lists of sources of prebiotics, research shows that many bacteria proliferate as a result of our eating these foods. Eat more of these foods and other foods rich in fiber to give the beneficial bacteria present in your gut a boost.

◊ The Prebiotics: FOS and Inulin

Two of the main prebiotics, FOS and inulin, have been heavily commercialized and are added to various food products and supplements.

While they are indeed beneficial, if you are eating a diet rich in fruit, vegetables, nuts, seeds, and legumes, they are of questionable importance. This is especially true if you regularly eat a range of fermented foods that contain both probiotics and prebiotics to feed the beneficial microbes, encouraging their proliferation in your gut.

If you choose foods or supplements that state: "contains FOS" or "fructooligosaccharides" or "contains inulin" on product labels, keep in mind that "oligosaccharides" are simply sugar molecules and "fructo" means that the sugars are derived from fruit. While these prebiotics certainly have merit, it may not be worth spending extra on products that contain them.

An Apple a Day Keeps Harmful Bacteria at Bay

While they have not garnered the attention of exotic superfoods, apples are superfoods in their own right when it comes to gut health and warrant greater inclusion in our diets for many reasons.

A Japanese study found that eating two apples daily for as little as two weeks significantly increases many Lactobacilli and Bifidobacteria bacteria in the gut, which greatly supports gut health.[22]

In another study, apples have been shown to significantly alter the amounts of the bacteria *Clostridiales* and *Bacteroides* in the large intestine, conferring gastrointestinal health benefits.[23] In addition to reducing the likelihood of suffering from one of these serious infectious conditions, simply reducing these harmful microbes also gives beneficial microbes a greater chance of survival in your gut.

Additionally, because apples are a good source of a special form of fiber known as pectin, which acts as a prebiotic that feeds beneficial microbes, apples are an excellent food to include in your diet on a daily basis to boost probiotics in your gut.

Their magnesium content also helps to relax intestinal tissues, supporting healthy eliminative processes and healthier gut tissue.

Surprising Food Boosts Beneficial Gut Bacteria

Who doesn't love a delicious plate of pasta with tomato sauce? I love a bowl full of brown rice noodles smothered in homemade tomato sauce made from my organic tomatoes fresh from my garden. Taste alone is enough reason to love this Italian favorite. But, now there is more reason than ever to love a plate full of spaghetti with plentiful amounts of tomato sauce—the pureed red fruit provides a serious boost to gut health.

It turns out that probiotics love tomatoes as much as we do, according to research published in the *Journal of Functional Foods,* which found that microbes (the good kind) enjoy a plate of spaghetti. Okay, maybe not a plate of pasta, but they love nibbling on the tomatoes from which the sauce originates. And to thank us for the feast, they multiply.

That's because tomatoes act as *pre*biotics thereby giving beneficial bacteria food from which to grow their numbers. The end result is a healthier gut and better overall health since gut health is linked to a growing list of health benefits, including: improved immunity to superbugs, reduced allergies, less pain and inflammation, better moods, and much more.

The researchers assessed both raw and cooked tomatoes under digestive conditions alongside the probiotic known as *Lactobacillus reuteri* (*L. reuteri*), which is known for its gut-health-promoting effects. While both raw and cooked tomatoes offered gut health benefits, the researchers found that the benefits of cooked tomatoes were greater than their raw counterparts at boosting *L. reuteri*.[24]

How can you benefit from the research? Add more tomatoes and tomato sauce to your diet. Avoid white pasta or egg noodles, which are also typically made from refined white flour and can actually encourage the growth of harmful bacteria or yeasts in the intestines and may thwart your best efforts. Instead, choose whole grain and gluten-free pasta options such as brown rice, quinoa, or even pasta made from legumes like black beans, which is also delicious.

Cooked tomatoes increased the benefits of *L. reuteri* more than raw tomatoes, but the addition of more tomatoes of either the cooked or raw varieties should ultimately be the goal.

Choose only organic tomatoes, since tomatoes are heavily sprayed with harmful microbes, and some of these pesticides have been linked to harmful imbalances of gut microbes. In other words, chemically sprayed tomatoes can throw off the delicate microbial balance in your gut.

As an added bonus, add a splash of olive oil to your tomato sauce toward the end of the cook time since it will boost up the absorption of the potent antioxidant found in tomatoes, known as lycopene. Enjoy your delicious plate of pasta knowing that the beneficial microbes who share your space will be enjoying it as much as you.

How Walnuts Transform Your Gut Health and Microbiome

From brain health to anti-inflammatory compounds, to anticancer compounds and more, walnuts are increasingly being touted as under-appreciated superfoods that we should elevate to a higher status in our diet, thanks to a growing body of research.

While all of these health benefits are reason enough to love walnuts, exciting research shows that walnuts can even transform the health of our microbiome, which may actually be reason for walnuts' amazing health benefits.

As you may recall from our earlier discussions, a microbiome is the sum of all the microbes that reside in or on our bodies. Every person or other living beings have a microbiome that is a unique signature of that particular being. In other words, no two people have the same microbiome. It is like our microbial fingerprint.

Our microbiomes change over time, depending on the foods we eat, the drugs we take (antibiotics destroy many beneficial bacteria), and other lifestyle factors. Now, research published in the *Journal of Nutrition* also found that walnuts can have a profoundly beneficial effect on our microbiome.[25]

Researchers at the University of Illinois at Urbana-Champaign explored how walnuts affect the trillions of mostly beneficial gut microbes in humans. Study participants ate walnuts or no walnuts as part of their diet for three weeks. Researchers analyzed fecal and blood samples before and at the end of the three-week study to determine if there had been any changes.

They found an increase in three types of bacteria: *Faecalibacterium, Roseburia,* and *Clostridium*—all of which secrete a compound known as butyrate when they are exposed to walnuts. Butyrate has been linked to improvements in bowel health. Higher levels of *Faecalibacterium* have been linked to reductions in inflammation as well as improvements in insulin sensitivity—a factor that improves blood sugar levels and suggests that walnuts may have benefits for diabetics and those people suffering from blood sugar imbalances.

It is too soon to know whether *Faecalibacterium* are probiotics, but the researchers say that the evidence suggests that is the case. However, don't go looking for these bacterial helpers in your probiotic supplement as you won't find them there. To reap the benefits of this bacteria, you'll simply need to eat more walnuts. Of course, avoid them if you're allergic to tree nuts.

If you're like most people you're probably already confessing your hatred of walnuts. Your face may already be wincing at the thought of eating more of the nuts. As a former walnut-hater, I can tell you that you may not actually hate high-quality, fresh walnuts. In my experience, most of the walnuts found in grocery stores, particularly those in the baking ingredients aisle, are old and rancid. When walnuts go rancid they get a disgustingly bitter taste that leaves an unpleasant film in the mouth.

Fresh, raw walnuts are a taste sensation. They have a delightfully buttery texture and mild, sweet flavor. They make a great addition to salads (especially over a bed of baby spinach with a fruity or citrus vinaigrette), or atop yogurt or bowl of fruit. My sister makes a delicious quinoa salad with fresh, chopped walnuts, sundried tomatoes, and a garlicky vinaigrette. I throw in a handful or two along with fresh or frozen fruit and almond milk for my morning smoothie.

And perhaps my favorite way to use walnuts: I make a delightful vegan, fermented cheese by soaking a cup of walnuts in half a cup of water, along with the contents of a capsule of probiotics, and leave them overnight to culture. Then, I blend them with any flavor additions and a bit of coconut oil until it forms a smooth cheese. Check out my book *The Cultured Cook* to learn how to make probiotic-rich walnut cheese and to find the recipe.

Feeding beneficial microbes helps to boost their ability to proliferate. Adding at least two servings of key prebiotic foods like apples, Jerusalem artichokes, leeks, onions, garlic, chicory root, asparagus, bananas, dandelions, endive, radicchio, burdock, tomatoes, and walnuts, you'll ensure the beneficial microbes have the food they need to proliferate, further helping to eliminate harmful microbes.

For Step Four, it's important to eat at least one food every day to feed the probiotics in your gut. Doing so makes the best use of the beneficial bacteria and yeasts you already have present in your gut, which helps them to fight off harmful infectious microbes. Additionally, giving them their favorite foods also helps to ensure that any probiotic supplements you take will go further by potentially magnifying the numbers of microbes. And, if that wasn't good enough: you'll also help to boost the probiotics naturally found in any fermented foods you eat. As you can see, feeding the microbes you have, take, or ingest has the potential for you to reap great health rewards.

It doesn't have to be a lot of each of the food but it is a good idea to give them some of the foods mentioned above on a daily basis.

⟶ STEP FIVE ⟵
Water Your Beneficial Microbes

You're not the only one that needs water. Make sure you're drinking plenty of water because, like you, beneficial microbes need water to function. This is also true if you're ingesting fermented foods or taking probiotic supplements since you're boosting their population in your gut at that time, and they'll need more water to perform their functions.

This is especially true when taking probiotic supplements. It is important to drink plenty of water when taking them. Probiotics found in capsules or powders are basically inert until they are mixed with water, and like humans, probiotics need water for their survival. The water rehydrates the bacteria, allowing them to become active so they can perform their many health-building functions. Once rehydrated, they work their magic in your intestines to help maintain or restore great health.

Additionally, you need sufficient water to ensure healthy bowel movements that transport harmful microbes, and those that have been destroyed in battle with healthy microbes, out of your body.

Drink at least one-half quart or one-half liter of water for every fifty pounds of weight you're carrying, up to three quarts or liters daily, to ensure beneficial microbes have the water they need and that harmful microbes are more readily removed from the body as they are destroyed. Regarding the latter, water and fiber are both necessary to form healthy stools that remove harmful microbes in bowel movements. I know this seems like a lot of water (because it is!), but it is important to help eliminate harmful microbes from the body.

Ideally, drink unchlorinated water or water that has been filtered, which can even be done through an inexpensive water pitcher that filters chlorine and prevents the killing of beneficial microbes.

Wherever possible, it's best to drink unchlorinated water since chlorine indiscriminately kills bacteria, good or bad. There are many inexpensive water filters or filtration systems available that remove most chlorine from drinking water. If you make your own fermented foods, you'll also need to use unchlorinated water to obtain the best results. Learn more about making your own fermented foods in my book *The Cultured Cook*.

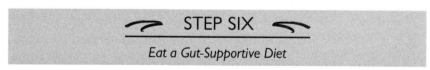

STEP SIX

Eat a Gut-Supportive Diet

All gut bacteria and yeasts, good or bad, fight for space and nutrients in your intestines. In your bowels, that means they battle each other for attachment to your intestinal walls and for the nutrients you provide them with through the foods you eat. Eat a lousy diet and you'll feed the harmful bacteria, but if you eat a diet full of fiber and natural pre-biotics and a small amount of healthy sugars from fruit, you'll feed the beneficial ones. We've all heard the old adage, "you are what you eat," and when it comes to gut and immune health, the sentiment could not be truer.

Research shows that the health of your gut is significantly influenced by what you eat. A study published in *American Society for Microbiology (ASM) Journal* evaluated 15,096 fecal samples provided by 11,336 people and found some interesting facts about gut health and the microbiome, including:

1. Plant-based diets produce the most diverse microbiomes. Diverse microbiomes seem to confer health benefits.
2. Eating more than thirty types of plant foods weekly yields the most diverse microbiome.
3. There is a lower incidence of bacterial resistance in those who eat the greatest variety of plant foods weekly.
4. People who ate more than thirty types of plant foods weekly had less resistance to antibiotics.
5. A connection between gut health and mental health.[26]

Does that mean you need to swear off all poultry, eggs, fish, or meat? No, of course not. If you prefer a vegan or vegetarian diet, that's your choice. Plant-based does not mean plant-exclusive; it means that the bulk of a person's diet is plant foods like vegetables, fruits, nuts, grains, seeds, and legumes. There are many ways to boost the variety of plant-based foods you consume and to move your diet to a more plant-based choice. I've included some ways to help you get started in the text box that follows.

Here are some suggestions to help you get started, but keep in mind that your choices should be whole foods, not heavily processed ones:

1. One day a week or more eat only plant foods. Start with Meatless Mondays but also be sure to make plant foods the focal part of your meals every day.

2. The next time you pass by that odd-looking fruit or vegetable in the produce section of your grocery store, add it to your cart. It's easy enough to find recipes for lesser-known foods using a quick internet search. And, most importantly, add the food to your diet.

3. Instead of just snacking on almonds or another nut, branch out to try Brazil nuts, cashews, hazelnuts, pecans, pistachios, and of course, walnuts. Choose raw, unsalted varieties.

4. Rather than just adding a can of kidney beans to your soup, stew, or chili, opt for bean varieties you are less familiar with. That could include chickpeas, lentils, pinto beans, Romano beans, black beans, navy beans, and others.

5. The next time a snack attack strikes, choose a piece of fruit or a bowl of mixed berries, or some fermented pickles instead of chips or chemical-laden "buttery" popcorn.

While this study didn't specifically explore the effects of fiber, we already know that some fiber is used as food for beneficial microbes while other fiber assists in removing destroyed harmful microbes from the gut. Either way, a high-fiber diet helps boost great gut health.

Of course, you'll get lots of fiber if you follow the dietary guidelines we just discussed, but to help you make sure you're getting 35 grams daily, here are some of the best fiber options.

Top Forty Whole Food Sources of Fiber

Getting enough fiber in your diet is critical to great gut health but goes far beyond that. Most nutrition experts recommend trying to get at least 35 grams of fiber daily. Here are some of the best fiber-rich whole foods. You may notice that I excluded gluten-containing grains in the list below. That's because they can be inflammatory to the gut, particularly in some people with other gut-health issues, so it is best for most people to avoid them.

Beans and Legumes: Few foods can compare with beans when it comes to fiber. If you're not already striving to get a cup of beans into your daily diet, now might be a good time. Here is the number of grams of fiber per cup of cooked beans:

Adzuki beans 17 gm	Kidney beans 16 gm
Black beans 15 gm	Lentils 16 gm
Garbanzo beans	Navy beans 19 gm
(chickpeas) 12 gm	Pinto beans 15 gm

Nuts: Nuts are an excellent fiber-rich whole food, provided you eat raw, unsalted ones found in the refrigerator section of your natural food store. Because they contain volatile oils, most nuts sold elsewhere have often been overheated during processing or exposed to excessive amounts of heat during storage, resulting in rancid oils. I haven't included peanuts because they are especially vulnerable to aflatoxins during storage—a type of mold that is inflammatory to the gut and damaging to the body; however, if you have access to a fresh source of peanuts, they may be fine. Here are some of the nuts highest in fiber per one ounce serving:

Almonds 4 gm	Pine nuts 12 gm
Brazil nuts 12 gm	Pistachios 3 gm
Cashews 1 gm	Walnuts 2 gm

Seeds: Most people rarely give seeds a second thought, yet the right kinds of seeds, like those listed below, are powerhouses of healthy fats, protein, and, of course, fiber. Since seeds tend to be used in different ways and in different quantities, I've listed the serving size followed by the number of grams of fiber for them:

Chia (2 Tbsp.) 10 gm	Pumpkin seeds (½ cup) 3 gm
Flaxseeds (2 Tbsp.) 4 gm	Sunflower seeds (½ cup) 6 gm
Hempseeds (2 Tbsp.) 2 gm	Sesame seeds (¼ cup) 4 gm

Berries: Not only do berries taste great, but they also tend to be high in fiber. The grams of fiber listed is per one cup of fresh or frozen berries. Here are some of the best high-fiber berries:

Blackberries 8 gm	Raspberries 8 gm
Blueberries 4 gm	Strawberries 3 gm
Elderberries 10 gm	

Whole Grains: Because many people suffer from gluten sensitivities, I've listed the top whole, gluten-free, high-fiber grains (the number of grams of fiber is per cup of cooked whole grain):

Amaranth 5 gm	Millet 2 gm
Brown rice 4 gm	Oats 8 gm
Buckwheat groats 5 gm	Quinoa 5 gm

Leafy Greens and Squash: Some of the best vegetable sources of fiber include leafy greens and squashes. The amount of fiber is measured in grams per cup of cooked greens or cooked squash.

Collard greens 5 gm	Butternut squash 6 gm
Kale 2.6 gm	Hubbard squash 7 gm
Spinach 5 gm	Spaghetti squash 2 gm
Swiss chard 4 gm	Summer squash 5 gm
Acorn squash 9 gm	Zucchini squash 3 gm

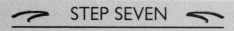

STEP SEVEN

Heal the Gut Lining

It's imperative to heal the lining of the intestines to prevent further infections and the release of toxic material into the bloodstream. There are multiple things you can do to help restore the gut lining.[27] But it's important to remember that it takes time to heal. It's not as simple as taking a drug to alleviate symptoms. It's necessary to begin the healing process at the source, not just alleviate symptoms.

Eating a low-inflammatory diet like the one we discussed, as well as incorporating probiotic-rich fermented foods and prebiotic-rich foods into your diet, as well as the other measures outlined in the previous six steps are critical to success. Additionally, it's important to avoid foods and lifestyle habits that thwart your best efforts. Cut back or eliminate concentrated sugars and alcohol to prevent candida and other microbes from overgrowing since their overgrowth and the byproducts of their proliferation can aggravate a leaky gut.

Limit or eliminate all processed foods as they usually contain excessive sugar, inflammation-causing fats, and toxic food additives, among other harmful ingredients.

The simple act of taking a fifteen- to twenty-minute walk after eating can be highly beneficial as well as it keeps the bowels moving while also oxygenating your blood. Your body's tissues require healthy, oxygen-rich blood to maintain their health or improve it.

Using herbs with a lengthy history of healing inflammation and the gut can also be helpful. Two of my preferred herbs for these purposes include aloe vera and licorice root.

Aloe Vera (*Aloe vera*)

Used for thousands of years, aloe vera is a powerful natural healing herb. When taken in its juice form, it has a reputation for being able to heal ulcers and ulcerations in the digestive tract while also gently assisting with bowel functions. Rich in amino acids, chlorophyll (the natural pigment that gives aloe its green color), enzymes (specialized proteins that assist the body with digestion), essential oils, vitamins, and minerals, aloe can help improve nutrient intake.

Because of its capacity to heal inflamed and wounded parts of the gut, aloe vera juice may help to heal the inflamed and excessively permeable gut tissue that is characteristic of a leaky gut.

Drink one-quarter cup of aloe vera juice, twice daily, ideally on an empty stomach. It is important to note that aloe vera juice is not the same as the gel, which is thicker and more concentrated. Avoid using "aloes" or "aloe latex" or products containing these components, as their bowel eliminative properties are quite strong. Also, be aware that aloe vera products frequently contain sugar, preservatives, and other additives, all of which should be avoided since they may actually irritate the gut or cause inflammation.

Licorice Root (*Glycyrrhiza glabra L.*)

Licorice root has a long history of use dating back to the Greek author Theophrastus who, as far back as 2,300 years ago, recommended the herbal remedy best known for its delicious taste we attribute to black licorice candy. The root has also been used for thousands of years in Chinese medicine. (Please note that Chinese medicine is not the same as traditional Chinese medicine, or TCM, which is a recent construct, although the latter is frequently incorrectly used by many authors and health practitioners.) Its popularity truly spanned the globe as it was used for thousands of years in the Middle East, and archaeologists even found a bundle of licorice root in Tutankhamen's tomb. It is a component of ayurvedic medicine (also called ayurveda), which is the ancient Indian system of medicine. The herb also has a lengthy history of use in North America among Native Americans and the First Nations of Canada, although it is not clear for how long the indigenous people used the remedy for the treatment of bronchial infections, coughs and colds, and urinary tract problems.[28]

One of a relatively small group of herbs known as adaptogens, which have the ability to improve overall bodily health by regulating functions as needed, as well as to give the body a boost to help it cope with physical, mental, or emotional stresses. In other words, adaptogens like licorice help the body adapt (like the name suggests) to just about any stress it encounters by increasing or decreasing the body's output of chemicals as necessary to achieve balance. That alone makes the herb an excellent choice for the immune system since it may help regulate immune activity and may even be helpful in the prevention of potentially deadly cytokine storms.

Licorice root is highly beneficial to the digestive tract. It has potent natural anti-inflammatory compounds, which is one of the reasons it is beneficial for the healing of the gut lining. Additionally, it helps eliminate toxic waste while soothing the walls of the intestines.

Licorice is a potent medicinal herb. As a result, it should be used with care; otherwise, it can have harmful side effects. Those with high blood pressure or kidney failure, or who are taking heart medications, should not use licorice. Licorice should also not be used in high quantities or for more than a few weeks at a time, without the guidance of a skilled herbal medicine practitioner or physician. Side effects are minimal if any, if daily intake of licorice's constituent glycyrrhizin, is kept below 10 milligrams. This ingredient has already been removed from most commercial herbal preparations of licorice root. You can tell by looking for the word "deglycyrrhizinated" on the label.

Follow package directions for the product you select. If you are using a licorice tincture, a typical dose is 1 to 3 milliliters, three times daily, for up to three weeks. To make a decoction, put half to one teaspoon of dried licorice root per cup of water together into a pot. Bring to a boil then reduce heat and let simmer, covered, for forty-five minutes. Strain. Drink one cup three times daily for up to three weeks. Do not use licorice if you're taking heart or blood pressure drugs, corticosteroids, diuretics, or monoamine oxidase inhibitors.[29] Because other drugs may interact with licorice, it's best to check with your physician prior to use.

7

The Guts for Super Immunity—for Life!

While the Seven-Step Plan for a Great Gut and Super-Powered Immunity often yields gut and immunity benefits in days or weeks and is intended to be continued for at least four weeks, it can easily become a powerful immune-strengthening plan for life. You may only need the antimicrobial herbal remedies periodically when dealing with harmful infections or when your health needs a boost, and indeed the herbs should not be continued for long periods of time—usually three to four weeks and then it's a good idea to take a break from them. The rest of the plan is perfect for long-term use and tends to work well to improve digestion, transform immunity, and strengthen overall health. But there are some additional strategies that are worth including in your life for super-powered immunity. In this chapter, we'll explore:

- how stress can impact your gut and immune system health;
- how adopting some simple stress-reducing strategies can have a big impact on your health; and
- how improving the quality (and in some cases) quantity of sleep you get can boost your immune health even more.

THE LIFESTYLE FACTOR THAT HARMS GUT HEALTH AS MUCH AS JUNK FOOD

We all know that junk food is harmful to our health. I recall some friends many years ago referring to cola as "gut rot" and probably for good reason. We all know that eating a diet high in junk foods like soda, chips, candy bars, and fast foods will likely result in poor health. Yet few people realize that stress can be just as damaging to our gut health as junk food.

In a study published in the medical journal *Scientific Reports,* researchers found that stress had a significant effect on changing gut microbes among female animals but not on males. The researchers explored the connections between obesity, stress, mood disorders, and gut microbes. They found that the gut microbes of lean female animals changed when they experienced stress to more closely resemble the varieties and volumes of microbes in obese mice. The male animals did not experience the same effect from stress. It was not clear why. As an aside: while stress did not have the adverse effect on males' gut microbes, the researchers also explored the effects of a high-fat diet on both female and male mice, and they found that males were more likely to experience anxiety caused by eating a high-fat diet.[1] But I digress.

The study showed us that stress, particularly when it becomes chronic or long-term stress, can throw off our intestinal microbial balance. And we probably didn't need the study to know that it is imperative that we find coping methods for reducing stress in our lives.

Obviously, there are many ways to help manage stress or at least reduce its impact on our lives. Some will undoubtedly be more effective than others depending on your unique personality, but here are a few of my favorites: deep breathing, venting with a trusted friend, changing jobs if it is job-related stress, changing homes if housing costs exceed our budget, meditation, exercise, getting out into nature, or getting into a hot bath with some stress-alleviating essential oils like lavender or vetiver. Learn more about how to reduce stress hormones with essential oils in my book *Essential Oils for Hormone Bliss.*

Of course, you may have other favorite ways to alleviate stress or lessen its impact. I love to take walks on my forest trails, spend time cooking some of my favorite dishes, and crank up the music and sing at top volume. What works for me may not work for you. Find the best strategies for you and stick with them. Consistency is key when it comes to stress management, and obviously to lessen the effects of stress on your gut microbiome.

SLEEP YOUR WAY TO A HEALTHIER GUT (AND IMMUNE SYSTEM)

Everyone has experienced the effects of sleep deprivation at some point or another: fatigue, brain fog, memory lapses, general malaise, and of course, feeling run down and vulnerable to whatever infection is going around at the time. Most people don't give the loss of sleep too much consideration until the problem occurs on a regular basis and disrupts their ability to work or aggravates any health conditions they may have or leads to new health conditions. But research shows that not getting enough sleep may be doing more damage than most people might think.

In a study published in the medical journal *Molecular Metabolism,* researchers assessed healthy men of healthy weight to determine whether short-term sleep partial deprivation had any effect on their gut health. For two nights the men slept for just over 4 hours, between the hours of 2:45 a.m. to 7:00 a.m. For two additional nights the men slept normally, which in the study was defined as 8-1/2 hours between the hours of 10:30 p.m. and 7:00 a.m. They found that short-term sleep loss altered gut microbes in terms of the ratios between different varieties of bacteria. Some strains increased while others significantly dropped. The microbial changes were comparable to changes linked to metabolism disruptions.[2]

Additionally, the researchers found changes in insulin sensitivity, which is a factor in diabetes, metabolic syndrome, and obesity. Sleep deprivation, even for such short times, resulted in a 20 percent reduction in sensitivity to the hormone insulin. Insulin is a hormone that regulates blood sugar levels in the body. When blood sugar levels increase after eating, insulin ensures that the levels drop back down. When the body stops responding properly to insulin, the results can be damaging. When this impaired sensitivity to insulin happens over long periods of time, insulin resistance can result. Insulin resistance is a condition in which the body no longer responds properly to the natural compound secreted by the pancreas in response to sugars, which can result in blood sugar imbalances that can wreak havoc on any aspect of our health, including gut and immune health.

While the research was preliminary in nature, the effect of sleep deprivation on our gut microbial balance may help to explain why we feel so bad when we are deprived of our beauty rest. The study did not explore the longer-term impacts of sleep deprivation on the gut microbiome, but it is likely that chronic sleep loss would also yield harmful effects on the microbiome.

While the research continues, you don't have to lose more sleep worrying about the effects of sleep loss. Here are some simple strategies to help you improve the quantity (if necessary) and quality of sleep.

Six Strategies for Better Sleep

There are some excellent ways that can help you improve your sleep, some of which include:

1. Skip caffeine after 3:00 p.m.
2. Avoid eating at least 3 hours before bedtime to avoid uncomfortable digestive symptoms like bloating or heartburn that can make it difficult to sleep.
3. Try to go to bed at the same time each night to help your body adjust to this pattern. Try to maintain a regular relaxation ritual in

the evenings, which could involve stopping work at least a couple of hours before retiring and incorporating some of your favorite relaxing pastimes.

4. Avoid blue-light emitting technologies within a few hours of sleep. These include: computers, televisions, and cell phones. And make sure you keep them away from your head and body while sleeping, particularly if you use a cell phone alarm. Keep in mind that blue-light-emitting devices can interfere with sleep cycles and are best kept to a minimum a couple of hours before bed.

5. Have a bath before bedtime to help you relax; better yet, add some lavender essential oil to the bath. Lavender has been found to calm the entire nervous system within one minute, helping people to feel more relaxed and sleepier.

6. Stop working at least a few hours before bed.

It's probably no surprise that getting better sleep helps us to deal with the stresses that impact our lives as well, increasing its many benefits for our health.

Maintaining a healthy diet and lifestyle throughout life takes some effort, but the benefits to our gut and immune health are many, and they in turn help to boost our overall health so we feel at our best and more capable to greet our life with vitality.

Notes

INTRODUCING THE ESSENTIALS

1. G. Vighi et al., "Allergy and the Gastrointestinal System," *Clinical and Experimental Immunology* 153, Suppl.1 (September 2008): 3–6.

CHAPTER 1.
THE AMAZING GUT–IMMUNE SYSTEM CONNECTION

1. Revere Health, "A Brief Overview of the Immune System," Revere Health website, accessed October 1, 2021.
2. Institute for Quality and Efficiency in Health Care, "How Does the Immune System Work?" National Library of Medicine, National Center for Biotechnology Information website, accessed November 3, 2021.
3. Institute for Quality and Efficiency in Health Care, "How Does the Immune System Work?"
4. Institute for Quality and Efficiency in Health Care, "How Does the Immune System Work?"
5. Pritish K. Tosh, "What Are Superbugs and How Can I Protect Myself from Infection?" Mayo Clinic website, accessed November 4, 2021.
6. G. Vighi et al., "Allergy and the Gastrointestinal System," *Clinical and Experimental Immunology* 153, Suppl.1 (September 2008): 3–6.
7. Selma P. Wiertsema et al., "The Interplay between the Gut Microbiome and the Immune System in the Context of Infectious Diseases throughout Life

and the Role of Nutrition in Optimizing Treatment Strategies," *Nutrients* 13, no. 3 (March 9, 2021): 886.

8. "Vitamin," Oxford Dictionary online, accessed March 3, 2022.

9. Erika C. Claud and W. Allen Walker, "The Intestinal Microbiota and the Microbiome," in *Gastroenterology and Nutrition: Neonatology Questions and Controversies,* edited by Richard A. Polin (Saunders, 2008).

10. "Gut-Associated Lymphoid Tissue," The Free Dictionary–Medical Dictionary online, accessed March 1, 2022.

11. "Lamina propria," The Free Dictionary online, accessed March 2, 2022.

12. Susan York Morris, "Everything You Should Know about Lymphocytes," Healthline website, updated September 28, 2018, accessed March 3, 2022.

13. "Appendix," The Free Dictionary online, accessed March 2, 2022.

14. Claud and Walker, "Intestinal Microbiota."

15. Lindzi Wessel, "How Your Gut Is Controlling Your Immune System," Massachusetts Institute of Technology, Center for Microbiome Informatics & Therapeutics website, accessed March 2, 2022.

16. Wessel, "How Your Gut Is Controlling Your Immune System."

17. Samuel J. Spaiser et al., "*Lactobacillus gasseri KS-13, Bifidobacterium bifidum G9-1,* and *Bifidobacterium longum MM-2* Ingestion Induces a Less Inflammatory Cytokine Profile and a Potentially Beneficial Shift in Gut Microbiota in Older Adults: A Randomized, Double-Blind, Placebo-Controlled, Crossover Study," *Journal of the American College of Nutrition* 34, no. 6 (2015): 459–69.

18. Wessel, "How Your Gut Is Controlling Your Immune System."

19. Claud and Walker, "Intestinal Microbiota."

20. Mary Ellen Sanders, "Probiotics: Definition, Selection, Sources, and Uses," *Clinical Infectious Diseases* 46, supplement 2 (February 2008): S58–S61.

21. Matthew Trost, "The Secret, Social Lives of Bacteria: Exclusive Interview with Bonnie Bassler," TED Blog (April 8, 2009).

22. Donatella Comito, Antonio Cascio, and Claudio Romano, "Microbiota Biodiversity in Inflammatory Bowel Disease," *Italian Journal of Pediatrics* 40, no. 32 (March 31, 2014).

23. Philip C. Calder, "Nutrition, Immunity, and COVID-19," *BMJ Nutrition, Prevention, & Health* 3, no. 1 (May 30, 2020): 74–92.

24. Mary Ellen Sanders, "How Do We Know When Something Called 'Probiotic' Is Really a Probiotic? A Guideline for Consumers and Health Care Professionals," *Functional Food Reviews* 1, no. 1 (Spring 2009): 3–12.

CHAPTER 2.
DO YOU HAVE THE GUTS FOR SUPER-POWERED IMMUNITY?

1. A. Lyra et al., "Intestinal Microbiota and Overweight," *Beneficial Microbes* 1, no. 4 (November 2010): 407–21.

2. Manabu Tamura et al., "Effects of Probiotics on Allergic Rhinitis Induced by Japanese Cedar Pollen: Randomized Double-Blind, Placebo-Controlled Clinical Trial," *International Archives of Allergy and Immunology* 143, no. 1 (2007): 75–82.

3. Jiaming Liu et al., "Neuroprotective Effects of *Clostridium butyricum* against Vascular Dementia in Mice via Metabolic Butyrate," *BioMed Research International* (2015): 412946.

4. A. Lyra et al, "Comparison of Bacterial Quantities in Left and Right Colon Biopsies and Faeces." *World Journal of Gastroenterology* 18, no. 32 (August 28, 2012): 4404–11.

5. S. Hempel et al., "Probiotics for the Prevention and Treatment of Antibiotic-Associated Diarrhea: A Systematic Review and Meta-Analysis." *Journal of the American Medical Association* 307, no. 18 (May 9, 2012):1959–69.

6. E. Lonnermark et al. "Intake of *Lactobacillus plantarum* Reduces Certain Gastrointestinal Symptoms during Treatment with Antibiotics," *Journal of Clinical Gastroenterology* 44, no. 2 (February 2010): 106–12.

7. Mary Hickson et al. "Use of Probiotic *Lactobacillus* Preparation to Prevent Diarrhoea Associated with Antibiotics: Randomised Double Blind Placebo Controlled Trial," *BMJ: Clinical Research Edition* 335 (July 14, 2007).

8. ConsumerLab.com "Product Review: Probiotics for Adults, Children, and Pets," November 23, 2013.

9. X. W. Gao et al., "Dose-Response Efficacy of a Proprietary Probiotic Formula of *Lactobacillus acidophilus CL1285* and *Lactobacillus casei LBC80R* for Antibiotic-Associated Diarrhea and *Clostridium difficile*-Associated Diarrhea Prophylaxis in Adult Patients," *American Journal of Gastroenterology* 105, no. 7 (July 2010): 1636–41.

10. E. J. Videlock and F. Cremonini, "Meta-analysis: Probiotics in Antibiotic-Associated Diarrhoea," *Alimentary Pharmacology and Therapeutics* 35, no. 12 (June 2012): 1355–69.

11. G. Ayala et al., "Exploring Alternative Treatments for *Helicobacter pylori* Infection," *World Journal of Gastroenterology* 20, no. 6 (February 14, 2014): 1450–69.

12. Xandria Williams, *The Herbal Detox Plan* (Carlsbad, Calif.: Hay House, 2004), 83.

13. Gilbere, Gloria. "A Doctor's Solution to 'Plumbing Problems,' In Your Gut That Is!" *Total Health* 26, no. 1, 37 (February 2004).

14. "How Much Sugar Do You Eat? You May Be Surprised," New Hampshire Department of Health and Human Services website, accessed March 31, 2022. No longer available.

15. Leslie Ridgeway, "High Fructose Corn Syrup Linked to Diabetes," *USC News* (November 28, 2012).

16. N. Jaiswal et al., "High Fructose-Induced Metabolic Changes Enhance Inflammation in Human Dendritic Cells," *Clinical and Experimental Immunology* 197, no. 2 (August 2019): 237–49.

17. Mark A. Febrraio and Michael Karin, "'Sweet Death': Fructose as a Metabolic Toxin That Targets the Gut–Liver Axis," *Cell Metabolism* 33, no. 12 (December 7, 2021): 2316–28.

18. Michelle Moughaizel et al., "Long-Term High-Fructose, High-Fat Diet Feeding Elicits Insulin Resistance, Exacerbates Dyslipidemia and Induces Gut Microbiota Dysbiosis in WHHL Rabbits," *PLOS One* 17, no. 2 (February 23, 2022): e0264215.

19. Richard Agans et al., "Dietary Fatty Acids Sustain the Growth of the Human Gut Microbiota," *Applied and Environmental Microbiology* 84, no. 21 (September 21, 2018): e01525–18.

20. Michaeleen Doucleff, "Chowing Down on Meat, Dairy Alters Gut Bacteria a Lot, and Quickly," *NPR/WBEZ Chicago* (December 11, 2013).

21. Mehmet Salih Kaya et al., "In Case of Obesity, Longevity-Related Mechanisms Lead to Anti-Inflammation," *GeroScience: The Official Journal of the American Aging Association (AGE)* 36, no. 2 (April 2014): 677–87.

22. Nicola Wilck et al., "Salt-Responsive Gut Commensal Modulates T_H17 Axis and Disease," *Nature* 551 (November 15, 2017).

23. "Gut Bacteria Are Sensitive to Salt," HealthCanal website, accessed March 9, 2022.

24. "How Much Sodium Should I Eat Per Day?" American Heart Association website, accessed April 1, 2022.

CHAPTER 3.
PROBIOTIC-POWERED IMMUNITY: MEET THE FAMILY

1. *"Lactobacillus acidophilus,"* MicrobeWiki website, accessed April 1, 2022.

2. Aki Sakatani et al., "Polyphosphate Derived from *Lactobacillus brevis* Inhibits Colon Cancer Progression through Induction of Cell Apoptosis," *Anticancer Research* 36, no. 2 (February 2016): 591–98.

3. Smith Etareri Evivie et al., "*Lactobacillus delbruekii* subp. *bulgaricus KLDS 1.0207* Exerts Antimicrobial and Cytotoxic Effects in vitro and Improves Blood Biochemical Parameters in vivo against Notable Foodborne Pathogens," *Frontiers in Microbiology* 11 (September 24, 2021): 583070.

4. *"Lactobacillus casei,"* MicrobeWiki website, accessed April 2, 2022.

5. Enriqueta Garcia-Gutierrez et al., "Production of Multiple Bacteriocins, Including the Novel *Bacteriocin gassericin M*, by *Lactobacillus gasseri LM19*, a Strain Isolated from Human Milk," *Applied Microbiology and Biotechnology* 104, no. 9 (May 2020): 3869–84.

6. *"Lactobacillus gasseri,"* MicrobeWiki website, accessed April 2, 2022.

7. *"Lactobacillus plantarum,"* MicrobeWiki website, accessed April 2, 2022.

8. *"Lactobacillus reuteri,"* MicrobeWiki website, accessed April 2, 2022.

9. *"Lactobacillus rhamnosus GG* (ATCC 53103) and Its Probiotic Use," MicrobeWiki website, accessed April 2, 2022.

10. Y. Qin et al. "Identification of Lactic Acid Bacteria in Commercial Yogurt and Their Antibiotic Resistance" [in Chinese], *Wei Sheng Wu Xue Bao* 53, no. 8 (August 4, 2013): 889–98. English abstract available on PubMed.

11. Ruairi Robertson, "Why Bifidobacteria Are So Good for You," healthline website (July 25, 2017).

12. Viola Andresen et al., "Heat Inactivated *Bifidobacterium bifidum MIMBb75 (SYN-HI-001)* in the Treatment of Irritable Bowel Syndrome: A Multicentre, Randomised, Double-Blind, Placebo-Controlled Trial," *Lancet Gastroenterology & Hepatology* 5, no 7 (July 2020): 658–66.

13. *"Irritable Bowel Syndrome,"* Mayo Clinic website, accessed April 2, 2022.

14. *"Bacteroides,"* MicrobeWiki website, accessed March 11, 2022.

15. *"Campylobacter jejuni,"* MicrobeWiki website, accessed March 11, 2022.

16. "Rotavirus," MicrobeWiki website, accessed March 11, 2022.

17. David Groeger et al., "*Bifidobacterium infantis 35624* Modulates Host Inflammatory Processes beyond the Gut," *Gut Microbes* 4, no. 4 (July–August 2013): 325–29.

18. Mikkel Jungersen et al., "The Science behind the Probiotic Strain *Bifidobacterium animalis subsp. Lactis BB-12 *," Microorganisms* 2, no. 2 (March 28, 2014): 92–110.

19. Shunyu Yao et al., "*Bifidobacterium longum*: Protection against Inflammatory Bowel Disease," *Journal of Immunology Research* (July 23, 2021): 8030297.

20. Marco Toscano et al., "Effect of *Lactobacillus rhamnosus HN001* and *Bifidobacterium longum BB536* on the Healthy Gut Microbiota Composition at Phyla and Species Level: A Preliminary Study," *World Journal of Gastroenterology* 23, no. 15 (April 21, 2017): 2696–704.

21. Michael T. Murray and John Nowicki, "Probiotics" in *Textbook of Natural Medicine,* 5th ed., (St. Louis, Mo.: Elsevier, 2020), available online at ScienceDirect website, accessed April 4, 2022.

22. "*Streptococcus salivarius,*" MicrobeWiki website, accessed April 4, 2022.

23. "*Streptococcus thermophilus,*" MicrobeWiki website, accessed April 4, 2022.

24. Azita Azad et al., "Protective Effect of the Probiotic Bacterium *Streptococcus thermophilus* on *Candida albicans* Morphogenesis and a Murine Model or Oral Candidiasis," *Iranian Journal of Medical Sciences* 46, no. 3 (May 2021): 207–17.

25. Li Qing et al., "*Streptococcus thermophilus* Inhibits Colorectal Tumorigenesis through Secreting b-Galactosidase," *Gastroenterology* 160, no. 4 (March 2021): 1179–93.

26. Deidre Rawlings, *Fermented Foods for Health: Use the Power of Probiotic Foods to Improve Your Digestion, Strengthen Your Immunity, and Prevent Illness* (Beverly, Mass.: Fair Winds Press, 2013), 13.

27. "*Saccharomyces boulardii,*" MicrobeWiki website, accessed April 4, 2022.

28. Eva Pericolini et al., "Therapeutic Activity of a *Saccharomyces cerevisiae*-Based Probiotic and Inactivated Whole Yeast on Vaginal Candidiasis," *Virulence* 8, no. 1 (January 2, 2017): 74–90.

CHAPTER 4.
THE PRO-POWERED SUPERHEROES AGAINST COLDS, FLU, AND SUPERBUGS

1. Anna Berggren et al., "Randomised, Double-Blind and Placebo-Controlled Study Using New Probiotic Lactobacilli for Strengthening the Body Immune Defence against Viral Infections," *European Journal of Nutrition* 50, no. 3 (April 2011): 203–10

2. Brylee A. Haywood et al., "Probiotic Supplementation Reduces the Duration and Incidence of Infections but Not Severity in Elite Rugby Union Players," *Journal of Science and Medicine in Sport* 17, no. 4 (August 31, 2013): 356–60.

3. M. Popova et al., "Beneficial Effects of Probiotics in Upper Respiratory Tract Infections and Their Mechanical Actions to Antagonize Pathogens," *Journal of Applied Microbiology* 113, no. 6 (July 2012): 1305–18.

4. Raakel Luoto et al., "Prebiotic and Probiotic Supplementation Prevents Rhinovirus Infections in Preterm Infants," *Journal of Allergy and Clinical Immunology* 133, no. 2 (October 13, 2013): 405–13.

5. E. Guillemard et al., "Consumption of a Fermented Dairy Product Containing the Probiotic *Lactobacillus casei DN-114001* Reduces the Duration of Respiratory Infections in the Elderly in a Randomised Controlled Trial," *British Journal of Nutrition* 103, no. 1 (January 2010): 58–68.

6. John Heinerman, *Heinerman's Encyclopedia of Healing Herbs & Spices* (New York: Reward Books, 1996), 333.

7. Paola Mastromarino et al., "Antiviral Activity of *Lactobacillus brevis* towards Herpes Simplex Virus Type 2: Role of Cell Wall Associated Components," *Anaerobe* 17, no. 6 (December 2011): 334–36.

8. E.I. Ermolenko, "Inhibition of Herpes Simplex Virus Type 1 Reproduction by Probiotic Bacteria In Vitro" [in Russian], *Voprosy Virusologii* 55, no. 4 (July–August 2010): 25–28.

9. T. M. Liaskovs'kyi et al. "Effect of Probiotic Lactic Acid Bacteria Strains on Virus Infection" [in Ukrainian], *Mikrobiolohichnyi zhurnal* 69, no. 2 (March–April 2007). 55–63.

10. "Worldwide AIDS and HIV Statistics," Be in the Know website by Avert, accessed November 23, 2021.

11. Soghra Khani et al., "In Vitro Study of the Effect of a Probiotic Bacterium *Lactobacillus rhamnosus* against Herpes Simplex Virus Type 1," *Brazilian Journal of Infectious Diseases* 16, no. 2 (March–April 2012): 129–35.

12. Neetu Gautam et al., "Role of Multivitamins, Micronutrients and Probiotics Supplementation in Management of HIV Infected Children," *Indian Journal of Pediatrics* 81, no. 12 (April 24, 2014): 1315–20.

13. C. Rask et al. "Differential Effect on Cell-Mediated Immunity in Human Volunteers after Intake of Different Lactobacilli," *Clinical Experimental Immunology* 172, no. 2 (May 2013): 321–32.

14. Mariya I. Petrova et al., "Vaginal Microbiota and Its Role in HIV

Transmission and Infection," *FEMS Microbiology Review* 37, no. 5 (September 2013): 762–92.

15. Haihong Hu et al., "Impact of Eating Probiotic Yogurt on Colonization by Candida Species of the Oral and Vaginal Mucosa in HIV-Infected and HIV-Uninfected Women," *Mycopathologia* 176, no. 3–4 (October 2013): 175–81.

16. WebMD, "What is a Peptic Ulcer?" accessed March 29, 2023.

17. WebMD, "What is Gastritis?" accessed March 29, 2023.

18. Breno Bittencourt de Brito et al., "Pathogenesis and Clinical Management of *Helicobacter pylori* gastric infection," *World Journal of Gastroenterology* 25, October 7, 2019 no. 37: 5578–89.

19. Lucia Pacifico et al. "Probiotics for the Treatment of *Helicobacter pylori* Infection in Children," *World Journal of Gastroenterology,* January 21, 2014.

20. E. P. Iakovenko et al., "Effects of Probiotic Bifiform on Efficacy of *Helicobacter pylori* Infection Treatment" [in Russian], *Terapevticheskii Arkhiv* 78, no. 2 (2006): 21–26.

21. Y. Aiba et al., "Lactic Acid-Mediated Suppression of *Helicobacter pylori* by the Oral Administration of *Lactobacillus salivarius* as a Probiotic in a Gnotobiotic Murine Model," *American Journal of Gastroenterology* 93, no. 11 (November 1998): 2097–101.

22. M. H. Coconnier et al., "Antagonistic Activity against Helicobacter Infection in vitro and in vivo by the Human *Lactobacillus acidophilus* Strain LB," *Applied Environmental Microbiology* 64, no. 11 (November 1998): 4573–80.

23. Kathene Candace Johnson-Henry et al., "Probiotics Reduce Bacterial Colonization and Gastric Inflammation in *H. pylori*-Infected Mice," *Digestive Diseases and Sciences* 49, no. 7–8 (August 2004): 1095–1102.

24. A. M. Kabir et al., "Prevention of *Helicobacter pylori* Infection by Lactobacilli in a Gnotobiotic Murine Model," *Gut* 41 (July 1997): 49–55.

25. Dionyssios N. Sgouras et al., "*Lactobacillus johnsonii La1* Attenuates *Helicobacter pylori*-Associated Gastritis and Reduces Levels of Proinflammatory Chemokines in C57BL/6 mice," *Clinical and Diagnostic Laboratory Immunology* 12, no. 12 (December 2005):1378–86.

26. Martin Gotteland et al., "Modulation of *Helicobacter pylori* Colonization with Cranberry Juice and *Lactobacillus johnsonii La1* in Children," *Nutrition* 24, no. 5 (May 2008): 421–26.

27. Lucia Pacifico et al., "Probiotics for the Treatment of *Helicobacter pylori*

Infection in Children," *World Journal of Gastroenterology* 20, no. 3 (January 21, 2014): 673–83.

28. Mayo Clinic website, "Diseases and Conditions: Periodontitis."

29. Wim Teughels et al., "Clinical and Microbiological Effects of *Lactobacillus reuteri* Probiotics in the Treatment of Chronic Periodontitis: A Randomized Placebo-Controlled Study," *Journal of Clinical Periodontitis* 40, no. 11 (November 2013): 1025–35.

30. Hanna Sikorska and Wanda Smoragiewicz, "Role of Probiotics in the Prevention and Treatment of Methicillin-Resistant *Staphylococcus aureus* Infections," *International Journal of Antimicrobial Agents* 42, no. 6 (December 2013): 475–81.

31. Po-Wen Chen et al., "Synergistic Antibacterial Efficacies of the Combination of Bovine Lactoferrin or its Hydrolysate with Probiotic Secretion in Curbing the Growth of Methicillin-Resistant *Staphylococcus aureus*," *Journal of Medical Microbiology* 62, pt. 12 (December 2013): 1845–51.

32. Muya Shu et al., "Fermentation of Propionibacterium Acnes, a Commensal Bacterium in the Human Skin Microbiome, as Skin Probiotics against Methicillin-Resistant *Staphylococcus aureus*," *PLOS One* 8, no. 2 (2013): e55380.

33. Caitlin R. Musgrave et al., "Use of Alternative or Adjuvant Pharmacologic Treatment Strategies in the Prevention and Treatment of *Clostridium difficile* Infection," *International Journal of Infectious Diseases* 15, no. 7 (July 2012): e438–48.

34. John P. Mills, Krishna Rao, and Vincent B. Young, "Probiotics for Prevention of *Clostridium difficile* Infection," *Current Opinion in Gastroenterology* 34, no. 1 (January 2018): 3–10.

35. Pierre-Jean Maziade, Pascale Pereira, and Ellie J. C. Goldstein, "A Decade of Experience in Primary Prevention of *Clostridium difficile* Infection at a Community Hospital Using the Probiotic Combination *Lactobacillus acidophilus* CL1285, *Lactobacillus casei* LBC80R, and *Lactobacillus rhamnosus* CLR2 (Bio-K+)," *Clinical Infectious Diseases* 60, Suppl. 2 (May 15, 2015): S144–7.

36. G. Reid et al., "Oral Use of *Lactobacillus rhamnosus GR-1* and *L. fermentum RC-14* Significantly Alters Vaginal Flora: Randomized, Placebo-Controlled Trial in 64 Healthy Women," *FEMS Immunology and Medical Microbiology* 35, no. 2 (March 20, 2003): 131–34.

37. Cobi Slater, *The Ultimate Candida Guide and Cookbook* (Maitland, Fla.: Xulon, 2014).

CHAPTER 5.
FERMENTED FOODS: THE NEARLY FORGOTTEN WISDOM
OF OUR ANCESTORS

1. E. Guillemard et al., "Consumption of a Fermented Dairy Product Containing the Probiotic *Lactobacillus casei DN-114001* Reduces the Duration of Respiratory Infections in the Elderly in a Randomised Controlled Trial," *British Journal of Nutrition* 103, no. 1 (January 2010): 58–68.

2. E. Guillemard et al., "Effects of Consumption of a Fermented Dairy Product Containing the Probiotic *Lactobacillus casei DN-114001* on Common Respiratory and Gastrointestinal Infections in Shift Workers in a Randomized Controlled Trial," *Journal of the American College of Nutrition* 29, no. 5 (October 2010): 455–68.

3. Aarti Sachdeva, Swapnil Rawat, and Jitender Nagpal, "Efficacy of Fermented Milk and Whey Proteins in *Helicobacter pylori* Eradication: A Review," *World Journal of Gastroenterology* 20, no. 3 (January 21, 2014): 724–37.

4. Felix Aragon et al., "The Administration of Milk Fermented by the Probiotic *Lactobacillus casei CRL 431* Exerts an Immunomodulatory Effect against a Breast Tumour in a Mouse Model," *Immunobiology* 219, no. 6 (June 2014): 457–64.

5. Gabriela Pinget et al., "Impact of the Food Additive Titanium Dioxide (E171) on Gut Microbiota–Host Interaction," *Frontiers in Nutrition* 6 (May 14, 2019).

6. Marie Dorier et al., "The Food Additive E171 and Titanium Dioxide Nanoparticles Indirectly Alter the Homeostasis of Human Intestinal Epithelial Cells in vitro," *Environmental Science: Nano,* no. 5 (2019).

7. Héloïse Proquin et al., "Transcriptomics Analysis Reveals New Insights in E171-Induced Molecular Alterations in a Mouse Model of Colon Cancer," *Scientific Reports* 8 (2018): 9738.

8. Alex Weir et al., "Titanium Dioxide Nanoparticles in Food and Personal Care Products," *Environmental Science & Technology* 46, no. 4 (February 21, 2012): 2242–50.

9. Reham Samir Hamida et al., "Kefir: A Protective Dietary Supplementation against Viral Infection," *Biomedicine & Pharmacotherapy* 133 (January 2021): 110974.

10. Maria do Carmo Gouveia Peluzio et al., "Kefir and Intestinal Microbiota Modulation: Implications in Human Health," *Frontiers in Nutrition* 8 (February 22, 2021): 638740.

11. Hiroaki Maeda et al., "Effects of an Exopolysaccharide (Kefiran) on Lipids, Blood Pressure, Blood Glucose, and Constipation," *Biofactors* 22, nos. 1–4 (2004): 197–200.

12. H-L Chen et al., "Kefir Improves Fatty Liver Syndrome by Inhibiting the Lipogenesis Pathway in Leptin-Deficient ob/ob Knockout Mice," *International Journal of Obesity (London)* 38, no. 9 (September 2014): 1172–79.

13. Mamdooh Ghoneum and James Gimzewski, "Apoptotic Effect of a Novel Kefir Product, PFT, on Multidrug-Resistant Myeloid Leukemia Cells via a Hole-Piercing Mechanism," *International Journal of Oncology* 44, no. 3 (March 2014): 830–37.

14. Heeson Chon and Byungryul Choi, "The Effects of a Vegetable-Derived Probiotic Lactic Acid Bacterium on the Immune Response," *Microbiology and Immunology* 54, no. 4 (April 2010): 228–36.

15. V. K. Bajpai, S. C. Kang, and K. H. Baek, "Microbial Fermentation of Cabbage by a Bacterial Strain of *Pectobacterium atrospepticum* for the Production of Bioactive Material against Candida Species," *Journal de Mycologie Medicale* 22, no. 1 (March 2012): 21–29.

16. Andrew W. Nichols, "Probiotics and Athletic Performance: A Systematic Review," *Current Sports Medicine Reports* 6, no. 4 (July 2007): 269–73.

17. Roghayeh Shahbazi et al., "Anti-Inflammatory and Immunomodulatory Properties of Fermented Plant Foods," *Nutrients* 13, no. 5 (April 8, 2021): 1516.

18. Dawei Gao, Zhengrong Gao, and Guanghua Zhu, "Antioxidant Effects of *Lactobacillus plantarum* via Activation of Transcription Factor Nrf2," *Food and Function* 4, no. 6 (June 2013): 982–89.

19. Y. H. Ju et al., "Estrogenic Effects of Extracts from Cabbage, Fermented Cabbage, and Acidified Brussels Sprouts on Growth and Gene Expression of Estrogen-Dependent Human Breast Cancer (MCF-7) Cells," *Journal of Agricultural and Food Chemistry* 48, no. 10 (October 2000): 4628–34.

20. Jinhee Cho et al., "Microbial Population Dynamics of Kimchi, A Fermented Cabbage Product," *FEMS Microbiology Letters* 257, no. 2 (April 2006): 262–67.

21. Jai K. Kaushik et al., "Functional and Probiotic Attributes of an Indigenous Isolate of *Lactobacillus plantarum*," *PLOS One* 4, no. 12 (December 1, 2009): e8099.

22. Min-Kyung Park et al., "*Lactobacillus plantarum DK119* as a Probiotic Confers Protection against Influenza Virus by Modulating Innate Immunity," *PLOS One* 8, no. 10 (October 4, 2013): e75368.

23. Jin-Woo Jeong et al., "Anti-inflammatory Effects of 3-(4'-Hydroxyl-3', 5'-dimethoxyphenyl) Propionic Acid, an Active Component of Korean Cabbage Kimchi, in Lipopolysaccharide-Stimulated BV2 Microglia," *Journal of Medicinal Food* 18, no. 6 (June 2015): 677–84.

24. I. H. Jung et al., "*Lactobacillus pentosus var. plantarum C29* Protects Scopolamine-Induced Memory Deficit in Mice," *Journal of Applied Microbiology* 113, no. 6 (December 2012): 1498–1506.

25. Ryoko Katagiri et al., "Association of Soy and Fermented Soy Product Intake with Total and Cause Specific Mortality: Prospective Cohort Study," *BMJ* 368 (January 29, 2020): 1–12.

26. Haiqiu Huang et al., "Soy and Gut Microbiota: Interaction and Implication for Human Health," *Journal of Agricultural and Food Chemistry* 64, no. 46 (November 23, 2016): 8695–709.

27. Li-Xia He et al., "Dietary Fermented Soy Extract and Oligo-Lactic Acid Alleviate Chronic Kidney Disease in Mice via Inhibition of Inflammation and Modulation of Gut Microbiota," *Nutrients* 12, no. 8 (August 8, 2020): 2376.

28. Brooke Nicole Smith and Ryan Neil Dilger, "Immunomodulatory Potential of Dietary Soybean-Derived Isoflavones and Saponins in Pigs," *Journal of Animal Science* 96, no. 4 (April 2018): 1288–304.

29. Dong Hwan Kim et al., "Genistein Inhibits Pro-Inflammatory Cytokines in Human Mast Cell Activation through the Inhibition of the ERK Pathway," *International Journal of Molecular Medicine* 34, no. 6 (October 2014): 1669–74.

30. I. Made Arcana and Megu Ohtaki, "Multi-Target Models and Their Application to Data Analysis of Cellular Mortality Due to Radiation Exposure," *Hiroshima Journal of Medical Sciences* 54, no. 1 (March 2005): 9–20.

31. Francesca Gaggia et al., "Kombucha Beverage from Green, Black, and Rooibos Teas: A Comparative Study Looking at Microbiology, Chemistry, and Antioxidant Activity," *Nutrients* 11, no. 1 (December 20, 2018).

CHAPTER 6.
THE SEVEN-STEP PLAN

1. Michelle Schoffro Cook, *60 Seconds to Slim: Balance Your Body Chemistry to Burn Fat Fast!* (Emmaus, Pa.: Rodale Press, 2013), 184–88.

2. American Heart Association, "Advisory: Replacing Saturated Fat with Healthier Fat Could Lower Cardiovascular Risks," American Heart Association News website, accessed March 22, 2022.

3. Diuli A. Cardoso et al., "A Coconut Extra Virgin Oil-Rich Diet Increases HDL Cholesterol and Decreases Waist Circumference and Body Mass in Coronary Artery Disease Patients," *Nutricion Hospitalaria* 32, no. 5 (November 1, 2015): 2144–52.

4. Soheil Zorofchian Moghadamtousi et al., "A Review of Antibacterial, Antiviral, and Antifungal Activity of Curcumin," *BioMed Research International* (2014).

5. S. Ankri and D. Mirelman, "Antimicrobial Properties of Allicin from Garlic," *Microbes and Infection* 1, no. 2 (February 1999): 125–29.

6. David Hoffman, *Medical Herbalism: The Science and Practice of Herbal Medicine* (Rochester, Vt.: Healing Arts Press, 2003), 526.

7. Hena Rahman and Anil Chandra, "Microbiologic Evaluation of *Matricaria* and Chlorhexidine against *E. faecalis* and *C. albicans*," *Indian Journal of Dentistry* 6, no. 2 (April–June 2015): 60–64.

8. Christine Ruggeri, "Olive Leaf Extract Benefits Cardiovascular Health and Brain Function," on the Dr. Axe website (June 12, 2019).

9. Ok-Hwan Lee and Boo-Yong Lee, "Antioxidant and Antimicrobial Activities of Individual and Combined Phenolics in *Olea europaea* Leaf Extract," *Bioresource Technology* 101, no. 10 (May 2010): 3751–54.

10. Ruggeri, "Olive Leaf Extract."

11. Ruggeri, "Olive Leaf Extract."

12. Maria Fournomiti et al., "Antimicrobial Activity of Essential Oils of Cultivated Oregano (*Origanum vulgare*), Sage (*Salvia officinalis*), and Thyme (*Thymus vulgaris*) against Clinical Isolates of *Escherichia coli*, *Klebsiella oxytoca*, and *Klebsiella pneumoniae*," *Microbial Ecology in Health and Disease* 26 (April 15, 2015): 23289.

13. Shahab Qureshi, "Klebsiella Infections," Medscape website (June 10, 2019), accessed March 21, 2022.

14. Gloria Magi, Emanuela Marini, and Bruna Facinelli, "Antimicrobial Activity of Essential Oils and Carvacrol, and Synergy of Carvacrol and Erythromycin, against Clinical, Erythromycin-Resistant Group A Streptococci," *Frontiers in Microbiology* 6 (March 3, 2015): 165.

15. Amandine Brochot et al., "Antibacterial, Antifungal, and Antiviral Effects of Three Essential Oil Blends," *MicrobiologyOpen* 6, no. 4 (August 2017): e00459.

16. Hercules Sakkas and Chrissanthy Papadopoulou, "Antimicrobial Activity of Basil, Oregano and Thyme Essential Oils," *Journal of Microbiology and Biotechnology* 27, no. 3 (2017): 429–38.

17. Valentina Virginia Ebani et al., "Antimicrobial Activity of Five Essential Oils against Bacteria and Fungi Responsible for Urinary Tract Infections," *Molecules* 23, no. 7 (July 9, 2018): 1668.

18. Mohd Sajjad Ahmad Khan, Iqbal Ahmad, and Swaranjit Singh Cameotra, "*Carum copticum* and *Thymus vulgaris* Oils Inhibit Virulence in *Trichophyton rubrum* and *Aspergillus spp.*" *Brazilian Journal of Microbiology* 45, no. 2 (August 29, 2014): 523–31.

19. Mohd S. A. Khan, et al., "Sub-MICs of *Carum copticum* and *Thymus vulgaris* Influence Virulence Factors and Biofilm Formation in *Candida spp,*" *BMC Complementary and Alternative Medicine* 14 (September 15, 2014): 337.

20. James A. Duke, *The Green Pharmacy: The Ultimate Compendium of Natural Remedies from the World's Foremost Authority on Healing Herbs* (Emmaus, Pa.: Rodale Press, 1997).

21. Rita A. Trammell et al., "Evaluation of an Extract of North American Ginseng (*Panax quinquefolius L.*) in *Candida albicans*-Infected Complement-Deficient Mice," *Journal of Ethnopharmacology* 139, no. 2 (January 31, 2012): 414–21.

22. Kenji Shinohara et al., " Effect of Apple Intake on Fecal Microbiota and Metabolites in Humans," *Anaerobe* 16, no. 5 (October 2010): 510–15.

23. "What's New and Beneficial about Apples," Agricultural Business Information website, accessed April 6, 2022.

24. J. Garcia-Hernandez et al., "Tomato Antioxidants Enhance Viability of *L. reuteri* under Gastrointestinal Conditions while the Probiotic Negatively Affects Bioaccessibility of Lycopene and Phenols," *Journal of Functional Foods* 43 (April 2018): 1–7.

25. Hannah D. Holscher et al., "Walnut Consumption Alters the Gastrointestinal Microbiota, Microbially Derived Secondary Bile Acids, and Health Markers in Healthy Adults: A Randomized Controlled Trial," *Journal of Nutrition* 148, no. 6 (May 3, 2018): 861–67.

26. Daniel McDonald et al., "American Gut: An Open Platform for Citizen Science Microbiome Research," *ASM Journals* 3, no. 3 (May 15, 2018).

27. Harvard Health Publishing, "Putting a Stop to a Leaky Gut," Harvard Medical School, website (November 21, 2018).

28. David Winston and Steven Maimes, *Adaptogens: Herbs for Strength, Stamina, and Stress Relief* (Rochester, Vt.: Healing Arts Press, 2007), 171, 175.

29. David Hoffman, *Medical Herbalism: The Science and Practice of Herbal Medicine* (Rochester, Vt.: Healing Arts Press, 2003), 554–55.

CHAPTER 7.
THE GUTS FOR SUPER IMMUNITY—FOR LIFE!

1. Laura C. Bridgewater et al., "Gender-Based Differences in Host Behavior and Gut Microbiota Composition in Response to High Fat Diet and Stress in a Mouse Model," *Scientific Reports* 7 (September 7, 2017).

2. Christian Benedict et al., "Gut Microbiota and Glucometabolic Alterations in Response to Recurrent Partial Sleep Deprivation in Normal-Weight Young Individuals," *Molecular Metabolism* 5, no. 12 (October 24, 2016): 1175–86.

Index

About the Author

Michelle Schoffro Cook, Ph.D., DNM, is an international bestselling book author and a popular natural health blogger. She is also a doctor of natural medicine and acupuncture and holds numerous degrees and certifications in holistic nutrition and herbalism. An expert on building the ultimate immune system, she has discovered many super-immunity secrets along the way.

Michelle is a regular go-to health expert for some of the biggest women's magazines. Her work is regularly featured in *Woman's World* magazine. She has also been featured in *Woman's World* magazine's "Ask America's Ultimate Experts" column. She is frequently featured or consulted for her expertise for publications and sites like *First for Women, WebMD,* and *Reviews.com.*

The author of 25 books on natural health remedies, her recent book, *Pain Erasers: The Complete Natural Medicine Guide to Safe, Drug-Free Relief,* was selected as the "best new book" by *Woman's World* magazine, was the Gold Medal winner for a Foreword Indies Award in 2021, and was a Nautilus Book Award Silver Winner in 2022.

To learn more about her work and view her other books and publications, visit **DrMichelleCook.com.**

Other Books by the Author

*60 Seconds to Slim: Balance Your Body Chemistry
to Burn Fat Fast!*

*Be Your Own Herbalist: Essential Herbs for Health,
Beauty, and Cooking*

*The Cultured Cook: Delicious Fermented Foods with Probiotics
to Knock Out Inflammation, Boost Gut Health, Lose Weight,
and Extend Your Life*

*The Essential Oils Healing Deck: 52 Cards to Enhance Body,
Mind, and Spirit*

*Food Fix: The Most Powerful Healing Foods and How to Use
Them to Overcome Disease*

*Food Fix Recipes: The Most Powerful Healing Foods and
How to Use Them to Overcome Disease*

*The 4-Week Ultimate Body Detox Plan: A Program for
Greater Energy, Health, and Vitality*

*The Life Force Diet: 3 Weeks to Supercharge Your Health and
Get Slim with Enzyme-Rich Foods*

*The Phytozyme Cure: Treat or Reverse More than 30 Serious
Health Conditions with Powerful Plant Nutrients*

*Super-Powered Immunity: Natural Remedies for 21st-Century
Viruses and Superbugs*

*The Ultimate pH Solution: Balance Your Body Chemistry to
Prevent Disease and Lose Weight*

*Weekend Wonder Detox: Quick Cleanses to Strengthen Your Body
and Enhance Your Beauty*

BOOKS OF RELATED INTEREST

Super-Powered Immunity
Natural Remedies for 21st-Century Viruses and Superbugs
by Michelle Schoffro Cook, Ph.D., DNM

Cultivating Your Microbiome
Ayurvedic and Chinese Practices for a Healthy Gut and a Clear Mind
by Bridgette Shea, L.Ac., MAcOM

Restoring Your Intestinal Flora
The Key to Digestive Wellness
by Christopher Vasey, N.D.

Freedom from Constipation
Natural Remedies for Digestive Health
by Christopher Vasey, N.D.

Natural Antibiotics and Antivirals
18 Infection-Fighting Herbs and Essential Oils
by Christopher Vasey, N.D.

Overcoming Chronic Digestive Conditions
Release the Visceral Layers of Post-Traumatic Gut Disorder
by Nikki Kenward, CST-D, MCSS
Foreword by Eric Moya, RMT, CST-D, MS/Mfct

Optimal Digestive Health
A Complete Guide
Edited by Trent W. Nichols, M.D., and Nancy Faass, MSW, MPH

Holistic Keto for Gut Health
A Program for Resetting Your Metabolism
by Kristin Grayce McGary, L.Ac., M.Ac., CFMP, CST-T, CLP

INNER TRADITIONS • BEAR & COMPANY
P.O. Box 388
Rochester, VT 05767
1-800-246-8648
www.InnerTraditions.com
Or contact your local bookseller